Stronger links

A guide to good practice for children's family-based short-term care services

Edited by Vicky Jones, Christine Lenehan and Carol Robinson
for Shared Care Network

The POLICY PRESS

Shared Care Network

First published in Great Britain in 2000 by

The Policy Press
University of Bristol
34 Tyndall's Park Road
Bristol BS8 1PY
UK

Tel +44 (0)117 954 6800
Fax +44 (0)117 973 7308
E-mail tpp@bristol.ac.uk
http://www.bristol.ac.uk/Publications/TPP

ISBN 1 86134 165 2

Photographs used on front cover reproduced with the permission of Sally Greenhill
Cover design by Qube Design Associates, Bristol
Printed in Great Britain by Hobbs the Printers Ltd, Southampton

Contents

Acknowledgements

We are grateful to many people for their help in producing the original *Stronger links*. Firstly to the planning group, Roland Farley, Laura Farningham, Geoff Green, Chris Osborne and Clare Warne, for having suggested writing a good practice guide.

Thanks are also due to the six regional groups in England and the Welsh group for their contributions. The constructive advice offered by all members at the Shared Care Network 1995 Annual General Meeting was welcome, as were the considered comments from Brighde Boyle, Vida Douglas and the Birmingham Shared Care Scheme, Laura Farningham, Bernie Flanagan and the PACT team at York, Pauline Gowland, Pat Hayes, Peggy Maxwell, Chris Osborne, Ken Pugh, Philippa Russell, Isabel Southern and Suzanne Welsh. We are also grateful to members of the Shared Care Network Policy Group and to individual schemes and members who sent in material for the case studies and examples.

Thanks to Candida Smith and Beth Prewett for their work updating this new edition.

Thank you to Dave Worth of The Policy Press for the design and typesetting, John Carter for illustrations, Jenny Hanson for photography, Adrian Cuin for processing photographs and Dawn Louise Pudney and Karen Bowler of The Policy Press for copy-editing and proof reading.

Finally, we are grateful to the Department of Health for making the production of the first edition of *Stronger links* possible, and to the Epigoni Trust for supporting the publication of this revised edition.

Information on Shared Care Network

Shared Care Network (formerly Shared Care^{UK}) is the umbrella organisation for hundreds of family-based short-term care services in England and Northern Ireland.

The services around the country are organised into regional groups. The regional groups are a forum for support and information exchange and each group has representation on the Shared Care Network management committee. The management committee is made up of a balance of professionals and parents/carers from the following regions:

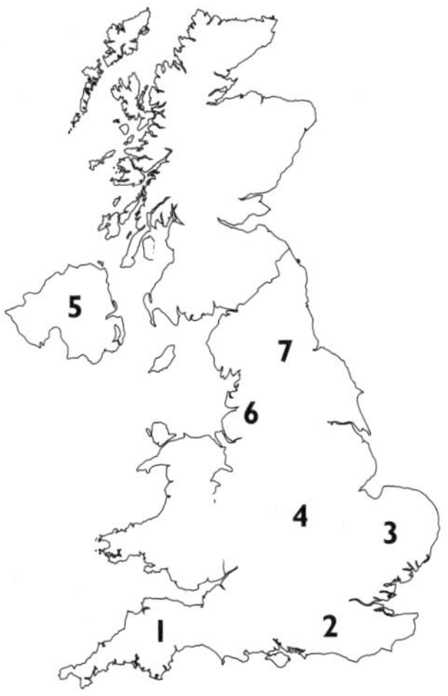

1. Shared Care South West
2. Shared Care South East
3. Shared Care Eastern
4. Shared Care Midlands
5. Shared Care Northern Ireland
6. Northern Shared Care
7. Shared Care North East

Membership information

There is a separate fee for regional membership and membership of Shared Care Network, although both are collected together for administrative ease.

Benefits of membership of a regional group

- Regular meetings for support, information and skills sharing.
- Outside speakers/workshops.
- Support for otherwise isolated workers.
- Discussion on practice and professional issues.
- Study days.
- Representation on Shared Care Network management committee.

Benefits of membership of Shared Care Network

- An entry in the Shared Care Network directory and free copy of the directory.
- Voting rights.
- Free copy of the Shared Care Network quarterly newsletter.
- Reduced rates for training events and conferences and direct mailing of information.
- Access to information and advice.
- Up-to-date information on new developments in family-based care.

Vicky Jones is the Shared Care Network National Coordinator. She has co-edited a range of publications for the organisation including *New horizons* (shared care and the needs of people with autism), *Towards a healthy future* (guidelines for the placement of children with complex health needs), and *Quality counts* (a review of quality assurance methods).

Christine Lenehan set up and now manages Barnardo's 'Families Together', a family-based short-term care service operating in partnership with the London Borough of Tower Hamlets. Christine is one of the co-editors of *Towards a healthy future* and has been an advisor to Shared Care Network since its inception.

Dr Carol Robinson is Senior Research Fellow at the Norah Fry Research Centre and is the leading academic in the field of short-term care in the UK. She has carried out extensive research in this area and has published widely. Publications include *Home and away: Respite care in the community*, *In safe hands?*, *Quality in residential short term care services* and *Growing up with disability*. Carol also acts as a consultant to Shared Care Network.

If you would like to find out how to join your regional group and Shared Care Network contact:

Shared Care Network
Norah Fry Research Centre
3 Priory Road
Bristol BS8 1TX
Tel 0117 946 7230 *or* 0117 928 9814 *or* 0117 973 1142

Introduction

Within England and Northern Ireland there are currently over 300 family-based short-term care services for disabled children. Most are based within local authority social services departments, although 21% are run by voluntary organisations (Prewett, 1999). Services are run in a variety of ways, although they generally agree that family-based care offers a better alternative to residential provision. The advantages identified can be summarised as follows:

- it enables users to develop real relationships with their carers and to develop wider social networks;
- the quality of care on offer is generally higher than that available in institutions and families feel less anxious about using a family-based service;
- family-based care is more flexible than residential short-term care, whether in a hostel or hospital;
- it is often a cheaper, more cost-effective way of providing high quality care than in other residential options.

The 1989 Children Act provided a basic set of standards to which services should subscribe. However, it did not provide detailed guidance on the various aspects of service delivery with which many service providers grapple on a day-to-day basis. As an umbrella organisation, Shared Care Network is often contacted by its professional members for advice and guidance of this type. This guide seeks to offer suggestions about the whole range of tasks that face professionals, to establish common standards and to clarify Shared Care Network's policy on a number of the most topical and thorny issues. *Stronger links* assumes that good practice will take place within the framework of the 1989 Children Act, and for this reason it is important to establish how disabled children and family-based short-term care is viewed under the Act.

The legislation

The 1989 Children Act represents one of the most wide-ranging and comprehensive pieces of childcare law ever passed in Britain. The Act not only sought to unify public and private law but also to apply to all children including disabled children. Disabled children are entitled to services because they fall into the category of children in need.

The law states that:

A child will be regarded as being in need if:

a) he/she is unlikely to achieve or maintain or to have the opportunity of achieving or maintaining, a reasonable standard of health or development without the provision for him of services by a local authority under this part (of the Act);

b) his/her health is likely to be significantly impaired, or further impaired without the provision of services;

c) he/she is disabled.

With regard to disabled children, the 1989 Children Act states:

Every local authority shall have services designed:

- to minimise the effect on disabled children of their disabilities; and
- to give such children the opportunity to lead lives which are as normal as possible.

Schedule 2, paragraph 2 of the Act requires local authorities to keep a register of children with disabilities, although there is no duty on parents to agree to registration.

These requirements should ensure that disabled children are seen as children first and disabled second and demand that local authorities give careful thought to how services are organised in order to maximise possibilities for children to be integrated into the wider community. Family-based short-term care services which provide opportunities for children to stay with ordinary families in the community exemplify how this can be achieved.

The Act, which places lead responsibility for the provision of services at the door of local authorities, is based on a number of key principles, which are highly relevant to family-based short-term care:

- the welfare of the child is **paramount**;
- **parental responsibility** rests with parents (even if a child is accommodated);
- services should be planned in **partnership** with parents;
- **prevention:** services should be provided in order to allow families to maintain their children at home;

- **consultation:** local authorities have duties to ascertain and take account of the wishes and feelings of children and parents in making plans for children.

These objectives were open to consultation and they may be subject to change over time.

Good practice in family-based short-term care services should be based on all these principles and in many instances the 1989 Children Act simply reinforced what was already happening prior to its implementation. However, there can be no doubt that finding effective ways of consulting some of the most severely disabled children remains a major challenge to all services.

In attempting to safeguard the welfare of children, the 1989 Children Act introduced two major changes for family-based short-term care by:

- treating all stays of 24 hours or more away from home as accommodation;
- requiring the people providing short-term care, lasting 24 hours or more, on a regular basis in their own homes, to register as foster carers.

Traditionally, family link services have been characterised by informality and flexibility and there was a great deal of anxiety among social workers that these changes would jeopardise the best features of them. While the 1989 Children Act regulations were a source of many difficulties, these were amended in August 1995 to take account of many of the concerns raised by Shared Care Network members and others.

The second edition of this guide comes at a time of significant change within social services. In recent years there has been an increasing concern about protecting vulnerable people of all ages following reports of widespread abuse of children living in care and adults living in residential settings. (See, for example, *People like us – Review of safeguards for children living away from home*, [Utting, 1997], and *The Independent Longcare Enquiry*, [Burgner, 1998].) At the same time, there is a greater emphasis on the efficient and effective use of resources, which is evidenced by the 'Best Value' initiative. To achieve greater efficiencies while enhancing safeguards requires reform and the government has issued a number of documents in which it sets out its proposals for reform of the NHS and social services. Of particular interest to shared care schemes are:

- The White Paper *Modern local government: In touch with the people* (DETR, 1998), which stresses that services should be delivered in the most effective, economic and efficient way possible.

- *Modernising health and social services: National priorities guidance 1999/00-2001/02* (DoH, 1999) (known as National Priorities Guidance), which outlines the aspects of health and social welfare services to be tackled in the next three years. This includes two relevant aims:
    - promoting the welfare of socially excluded children looked after by local authorities (this would include disabled children accommodated on shared care schemes); and
    - improving regulatory powers and duties to protect vulnerable adults and children from harm.

- The 'Quality Protects' initiative (1998) which is a three-year programme (attracting £375m of funding) that aims to remedy defects in the standards of care offered to looked-after children and those in need of support. It specifies national objectives for children's services and includes two full objectives and one sub-objective which are of special importance:

Objective 1: to ensure that children are securely attached to carers capable of providing safe and effective care for the duration of childhood.

Sub-objective 1.4: to increase the number of families of children in need supported by a series of planned short-term care arrangements involving for each child the same substitute (respite) carer.

Objective 6: to ensure that children with specific social needs arising out of disability or a health condition are living in families or other appropriate settings in the community where their assessed needs are adequately met and reviewed.

- The White Paper *Modernising social services* (DoH, December 1998) builds on all of the documents mentioned above and makes clear that a new, independent regulatory system will be established. This will involve the setting up of the Commission for Care Standards (CCS) with eight regional branches and the development of new national standards for regulation. Of particular interest is the recent publication of national standards and code of practice for foster care (UK Joint Working Party on Foster Care, 1999a, 1999b).

Such widespread changes are likely to preoccupy social services managers who are charged with the development of local action plans. It is therefore vital that those involved in shared care schemes are quick to capitalise on the positive endorsement of family-based short-term care found in the Quality Protects document by pointing out the benefits of their schemes, both in economic terms and as a means of countering social exclusion. However, such potential expansion should not be at the expense of high standards and it is vital that schemes keep sight of best possible practice. It is to be hoped that this guide will assist professionals in this task.

Who is this guide for?

This guide is intended to assist practitioners who are either setting up or running family-based short-term care services. It is also likely to be of interest to people who wish to use such services and to people who are in the position of purchasing.

How is it organised?

The guide is arranged in chronological sequence so that attention is given to publicity and access prior to chapters on preparation for carers and users. Each section of the guide begins with a box outlining the relevant current legal requirements or guidance. Thereafter each section focuses on specific ways in which services can enhance their practice. Wherever possible, examples of useful materials from services have been incorporated.

Glossary of terms

Throughout *Stronger links*, various terms are used interchangeably. These terms reflect their everyday use.

Family based-short-term care Short breaks Shared care	refer to an arrangement where a disabled child has a series of short pre-planned placements with a support family or carer. These stays take place with the same family/carer
Family link schemes/services Link schemes Shared care schemes Family-based short-term care services	all refer to services which organise family-based short-term placements for disabled children
Agencies Local authorities Voluntary organisations/agencies	refer to responsible authorities
Service/scheme coordinators Workers Practitioners Organisers Staff Link social workers (as opposed to child's own social worker) Professionals	refer to paid employees who run or work on a family-based short-term care scheme

Carers Hosts Support families Support carers Host carer Foster carers	refer to individuals or families who offer short-term care, in their own homes, to disabled children
Parents	refers to the disabled child's, natural parent(s) or guardian(s)
Carer's children	refers to the support carer's own children
Siblings	refers to the disabled child's brothers/sisters
The Act	refers to the 1989 Children Act

Publicity and recruitment

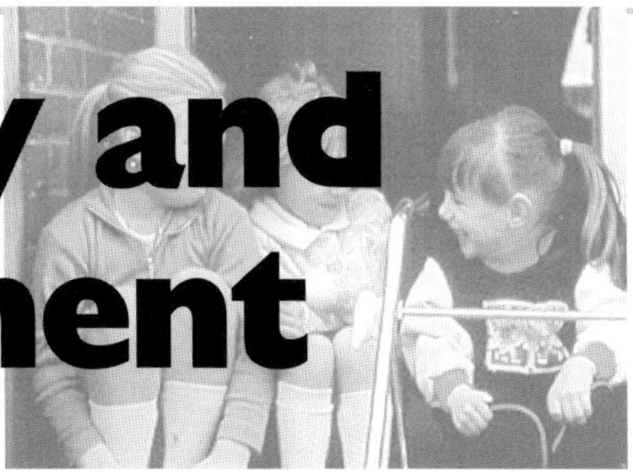

1

This section looks at:

- a variety of media for publicising services;
- effective ways of recruiting carers;
- using the media and other communication channels in recruitment campaigns;
- strategies for recruiting carers for children with autism, complex health needs and black carers;
- tips on making the most of the media.

Legislation and guidance

Publicity and recruitment campaigns should aim to reach all groups in the community, especially where there is or may be a need for foster parents from a particular racial, cultural or religious group. Local authorities are particularly required by paragraph 11 of Schedule 2 to the Act to have regard, in publicising and recruiting for the fostering service, to the different racial groups to which children in need in the area belong. (1989 Children Act Guidance and Regulations, Vol 3, Section 3.8)

Introduction

Short-term care services cannot provide care without carers. Service coordinators regularly need to recruit carers, advertise their services to potential users and generally inform the wider public about their existence. This section will therefore look at ways that this can be achieved.

Publicity and recruitment campaigns will almost certainly result in users as well as potential carers coming forward, because the campaign will have the effect of raising general awareness of the service. Therefore, material is best designed to inform both potential carers and users. If your service already has a waiting list you need to be prepared to explain the situation to parents.

Dear

Thank you for the referral on the above named child. I am sorry to say that it is not possible for us to undertake an assessment at this point in time.

We have a large number of children who are waiting for short-term care and very few carers who have space available.

We have, therefore, decided to concentrate over the next six months on a recruitment campaign for new carers, rather than undertake assessments on new children simply to put their names on a waiting list.

Do please, however, come back to us if this situation becomes urgent.

Yours sincerely

Some general points to bear in mind when thinking about publicity and recruitment:

- once a campaign is launched, be sure that fellow workers and administrative staff know about it so that telephone enquirers receive a good initial response. Enquirers only have one 'first impression';
- there are some periods during the year which are not good for recruitment, for example, before Christmas, around other major religious festivals and during annual holidays;
- it is worthwhile checking with the local authority whether it has a public relations person who can offer training to social workers in using the media so that you can get the most from your publicity campaign.

Publicity

All publicity should use accessible language, should be easily recognisable, that is, have identifiable logo/colour scheme/picture, and should be scheme-oriented rather than just social services publicity. It is also important to make sure that Family Link/Shared Care information is included in general fostering publicity. Information should be honest about remuneration and include an equal opportunities statement. One way of dealing with this would be to say something like: 'Carers are ordinary people from a variety of backgrounds, with or without a partner, young and old, with or without children, from all walks of life and who live in all kinds of housing' (see **Policy statements** section at the end of this guide for the Shared Care Network **Equal Opportunities Statement**).

Listed below are a range of possible media for educating the public about services. Some are much more expensive and time-consuming to produce than others, but it is important that a range of outlets are used to get the message across.

Leaflets

A single leaflet can cover both carers and users. Ensure that leaflets have a clear point of contact and that this can be easily updated should the contact change. Leaflets can be either multi-lingual (several languages on one leaflet) or translated into individual languages. Make sure you don't print too many as issues, language, addresses, and so on do change!

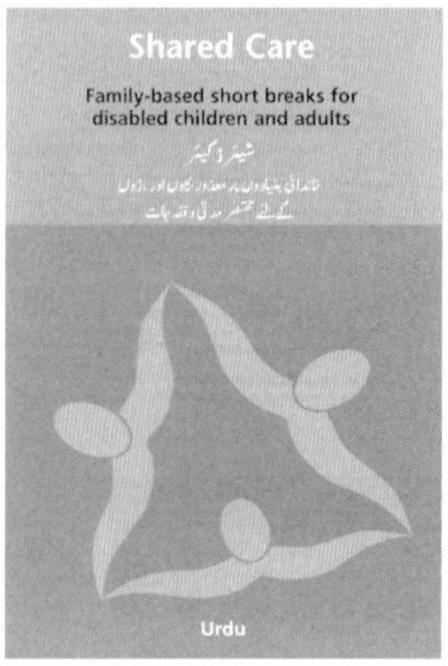

Shared Care Network has produced a lively eight-page leaflet on Shared Care/Family Link services which is aimed at both support carers and parents. The leaflet has been translated into Urdu, Gujurati, Punjabi, Bengali, Chinese and Vietnamese. Each A5 leaflet has a space at the end for services to insert their address and contact details. The leaflet includes details on:

- What is shared care?
- Who uses shared care?
- Who are the support carers?
- Are you interested in becoming a support carer?
- Do you have a disabled child or adult in your family?
- How can you find out more about your local Shared Care/Family Link scheme?

Multi-lingual leaflets may incur multi-lingual referrals, so make sure there are staff who can follow up the referrals. It may be useful to give a specific time slot for potential carers to phone in and ensure that the person staffing the phone during this time can speak the appropriate language.

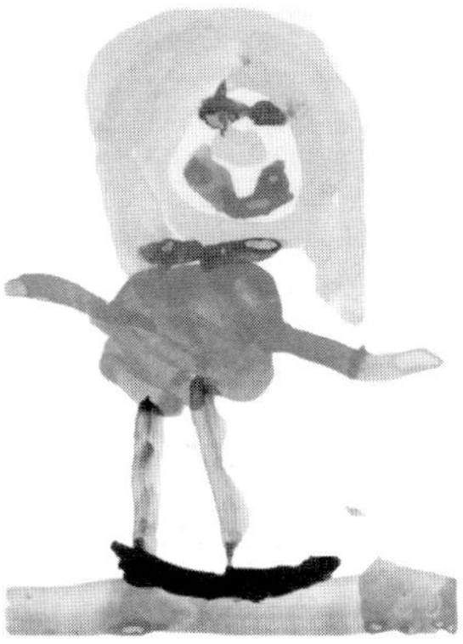

The photos used in publicity should reflect the communities being targeted. Some schemes use pictures drawn by children that can then be used on multi-lingual leaflets. The drawings shown here are examples taken from Northamptonshire, Mid Glamorgan and Nottingham Family Link schemes. These drawings promote a bright and positive image of the service. However, if the scheme is for both children and adults and you wish to use the same publicity for both, the pictures would not be appropriate. In this case use photos of children and adults or a drawing/graphic which is age-appropriate.

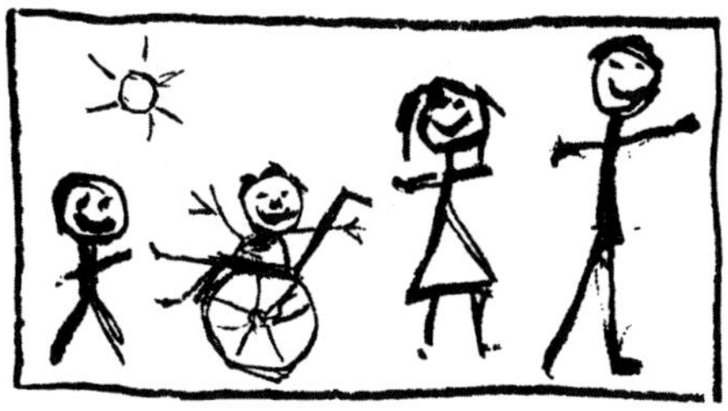

Research into the readability of charity leaflets (Sturmey, 1993) indicated that many leaflets were rated as dull and had little human interest.

When designing your leaflet make sure that you:

- use short words and sentences;
- refer to people, use quotations;
- address the reader directly;
- consider using a question-and-answer format;
- use photographs and line drawings to increase human interest.

Videos

Again, these can be a source of information for both carers and users. Videos can be expensive; to keep costs down consider:

- using local college media centres;
- producing a county-wide video;
- sharing costs with a neighbouring scheme.

Many schemes have produced their own videos. It may be worth considering buying one of these. There is a list of videos that are currently available at the end of this section.

Audio tapes

These should be produced in appropriate languages and also in simple language to allow children to understand what the service is all about. The advantages of audio tapes are that they are more accessible than the written word and cheaper to produce than videos.

Posters

Display in:

- libraries
- surgeries
- supermarkets
- shops
- buses
- community centres
- places of worship
- etc, etc

Do check that they are put up and visible.

Display stands

These can be scheme-specific or linked up with general fostering. Display stands can be put up in libraries, shopping centres, at fetes, fairs, and so on (some may need an attendant).

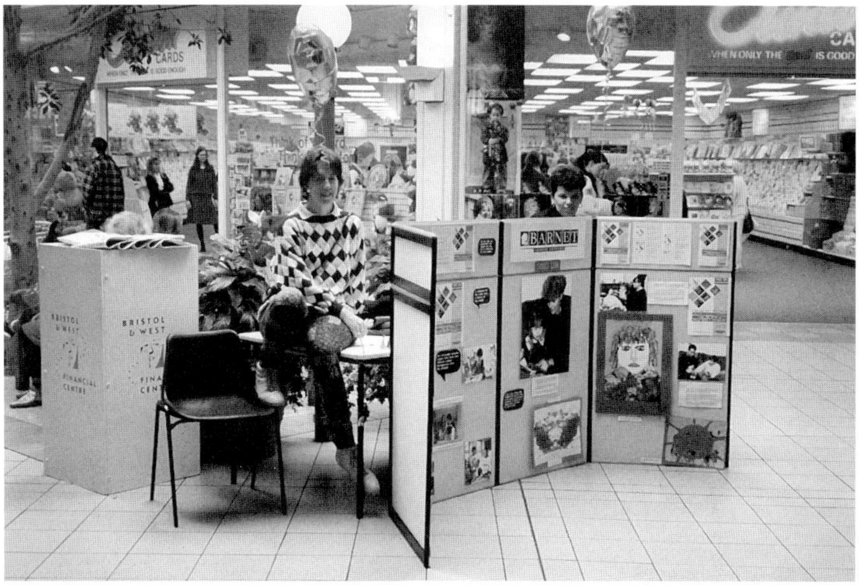

Flyers

Flyers can be distributed with local papers. These are cheaper and simpler than leaflets, but needed in large quantities. Many schemes have found it useful to contact head teachers for permission to give flyers to schoolchildren to take home. Other inventive ways in which schemes have publicised their services include adverts inside milk bills and wage slips.

Press

Adverts for general purposes or for specific children should be put alongside feature articles (see **Recruitment** on page 10).

The following advert used by a scheme in North Bristol was very successful in attracting a large response.

CAN YOU CARE?

A challenge and a reward

Caring people are wanted to help families with children who have physical and/or learning disabilities. By looking after children for anything between an occasional few hours, an overnight stay, weekend or part of the school holidays, you can offer the parents a much needed break and the children an enjoyable change.

Whether you are single, married, divorced, black or white, working or not working, we'd like to hear from you. We need all kinds of people to help all kinds of children and families. You will receive training, support and payment for the care given.

If you can help please contact:

Name ....

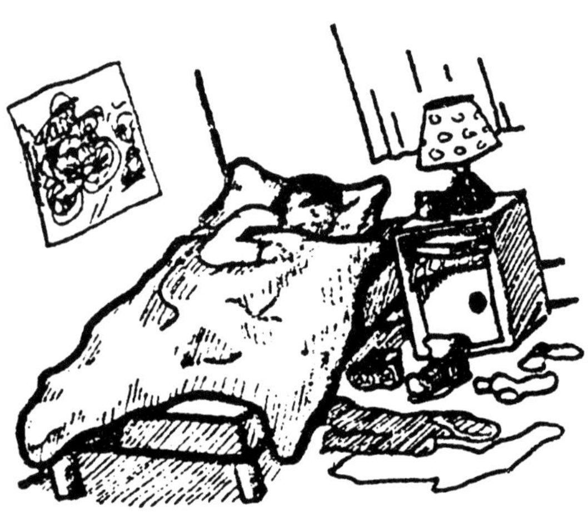

....

Address ....

....

....

Telephone ....

Reviewing your publicity

It is useful to conduct an annual review of publicity. Terminology, people and addresses change so bear this in mind when producing large numbers of expensive leaflets.

Recruitment – what works

One of the most effective ways of recruiting is word of mouth, and the following are ways of enabling this.

- Encouraging existing carers and users to tell their friends and supplying them with leaflets.
- Targeting those already 'in the business', for example, special schools (teachers, ancillary staff, parents).
- Childminders, social workers, health visitors, community nurses (for example, using the internal vacancy list).
- Asking parents if they know potential carers – some authorities will approve relatives, others will not. The 1989 Children Act regulations clearly state, however,

  ... possibilities for a child to be cared for within the extended family should have been investigated and considered as an alternative to the provision of accommodation by the responsible authority. However even when it has become necessary for the responsible authority to arrange provision of accommodation, placement with a relative will often provide the best opportunities for promoting and maintaining family links in a familiar setting. (1989 Children Act Guidance and Regulations, Vol 3, Section 3.33)

- Successful arrangements may be made with someone the child already knows. This could be with someone at arm's length from the family, for example, a school escort, nursing staff, dinner ladies, as well as family friends.
- Sitting and befriending services might also be usefully explored.

Recruitment campaign

A campaign is usually set up to launch a scheme, but can also be used for further major recruitment drives. Useful channels are:

The media

Make use of relevant local radio stations and newspapers serving a variety of sections of the community. The local authority public relations office will have information on relevant outlets. Local television is also a useful source of publicity.

For feature articles and interviews, enlist the help of carers and users in conjunction with professionals.

Recruitment for specific children in papers or radio can be fruitful if other avenues have been explored unsuccessfully. However, care must be taken to protect the child's interests. Use of pseudonyms and the careful substitution of factual information can help to protect the child and family's identity. Serious consideration should be given to whether it is in the child's best interest to provide a name and photograph. Parental permission would need to be obtained for use of photos and it is suggested that this should be used as a last resort. The advert opposite generated over 70 initial enquiries!

Could you help share the care of Gary, Milon and Delroy?

We need caring, responsible people who can welcome a child with a disability into their home for a weekend, holiday day care or one overnight weekend once a month and who can work in partnership with their parents.

Gary is five and very active. He's got lots of energy and likes to go to the park.

Milon is eight and uses a wheelchair. She enjoys company, music and outings.

Delroy is eleven. He is very agile and enjoys musical toys and going to the playground. You don't need any special qualifications, just lots of energy and understanding.

You can be any age, single or a couple, with or without children of your own. We will give you training, support and pay you an allowance.

Interested? Then get in touch today!

Either ring us on ....

for an information pack or write to us at ....

....

or attend our Open Session on .... at ....

Other communication channels

Other communication channels include:

- religious magazines;
- school newsletters;
- childminders' newsletters;

- the Diocesan information network;
- magazines of local charitable organisations such as The Rotary Club, The Round Table, Lions Club;
- Asian community magazines;
- obtaining a list of industries provided by the Chamber of Commerce.

Use the commercial world, that is, banks, building societies, supermarkets etc. Wherever possible ask organisations to distribute the information themselves!

Still having problems recruiting?

If you are having specific difficulties recruiting, contact schemes in similar areas such as inner-city or rural areas and see what has worked best for them. Wherever possible share your resources.

A useful publication with ideas for meeting the needs of children who are hard to place is *Why are we waiting?* (Robinson and Stalker, 1992).

It is clear that some groups of children wait longer for services than others. Suggestions for specific strategies for recruiting carers for children with autism, children with complex healthcare needs and children from minority ethnic groups follow.

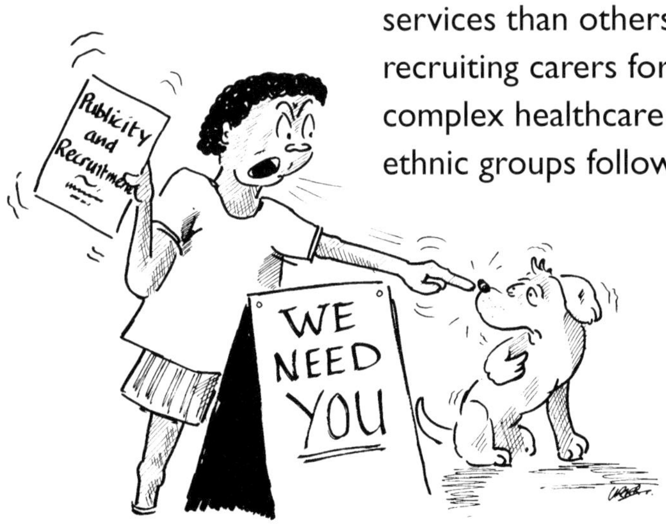

Recruiting carers for children with autism

Research indicates that children with autism are more likely to be on waiting lists for shared care than other disabled children (Donnelly and Horrex, 1995; Prewett, 1999).

Finding placements for children with autism may be more difficult because of the particular challenges they face when using short-term care services. High levels of noise, unfamiliar people and an unstructured atmosphere may cause anxiety and distress.

How can we encourage/recruit families to offer care to children with autism?

By recruiting carers in the usual generic way and giving information as part of their preparation, interested carers could be pinpointed at a relatively early stage.

Alternatively, carers could be specifically targeted by:

- approaching experienced carers;
- approaching professionals already working with people with autism or volunteers who have experience through play schemes etc;
- finding carers with similar interests to the child;
- bringing together potential carers and children with autism for play schemes or fun days. This may give them the confidence to offer a link to a child with autism;
- using salaried carers;

- working in conjunction with other agencies specialising in this field, for example, the National Autistic Society;
- reassuring potential carers that they will be given specific training on the needs of children with autism and continuing support.

Further information can be found in *New horizons*, a book produced by Shared Care Network (Jones et al, 1997), that offers useful advice for meeting the needs of children with autism who use shared care services.

Recruiting carers for children with complex healthcare needs

In recent years the number of children with complex healthcare needs has increased dramatically. This is due in part to advances in medicine, which mean that more children are surviving very premature birth and neonatal complications and those with degenerative conditions are living longer. Carers who offer short breaks to this group of children may be required to carry out certain routine clinical procedures, for example, giving feeds via a gastrostomy tube, suction or administration of rectal diazepam.

When recruiting for children with complex health needs, target health professionals, for example, nurses, health visitors, paediatricians. Carers offering breaks to children with complex health needs will be required to receive very specific training regarding the individual child's particular condition. For further information see *Towards a healthy future* (Servian et al, 1998).

Recruiting black carers

The following steps are suggested as a framework for a strategy to recruit black carers:

1 Being prepared

This involves considering three important issues:

A Commitment

Before embarking on a campaign to recruit black carers there has to be a full commitment from the agency and its staff. This is vital to the success of the campaign:

- staff need to be clear about the numbers of black families in the community;
- they should be aware that they have something to offer;
- white staff may need to reflect on their own attitudes towards other races and work through these in order to ensure that everyone is committed to equality.

B Creating a welcoming environment

The environment needs to be welcoming and respectful. A Barnardo's project in Tower Hamlets which has been very successful in recruiting black families displays its 'Statement of belief' clearly at the entrance to the office.

C Black staff

It is a bonus to have black staff on the team but a lack of black workers is not a reason to halt proceedings. If the agency does employ black workers, a word of caution. Do not expect your workers to be experts on all religions and cultures and, indeed, black issues generally. Many black workers feel pressurised and isolated when an agency employs them as a lone worker who is expected to solve all of the problems of attracting black carers to the scheme.

2 Identifying needs

What are the specific cultural and religious needs of the children to be placed? The needs of the children will influence the direction of the recruitment drive to specific groups or communities.

3 Planning and goal setting

The recruitment strategy needs to be carefully planned. What are the aims? How will they be achieved? Who is going to do what and by when?

For example, a goal may be to put together a list of community networks or agencies to contact as a starting point. Make sure that there is a clear time-scale for this and that all team members are allocated specific tasks.

4 Making communities aware of the service

Make links with the local communities. One of the most effective methods of recruiting carers is word of mouth. Work alongside community leaders or religious leaders in order to tell target groups about the service.

Building links with communities takes time. Simply going into a community and selling the service may not be the best way forward. There should be a two-way exchange where workers find out about the particular community and its culture. Investing time in building up relationships and trust at the outset will be worthwhile and pay off in the long run.

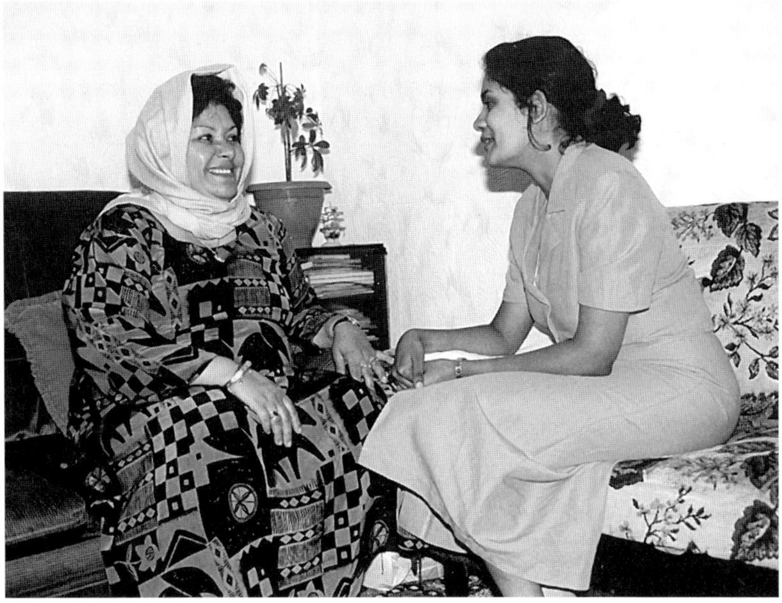

When it is appropriate involve established carers from the particular ethnic group being targeted so that they can present their experiences of being a carer.

5 Advertising

Once there are established links with the particular communities it should be possible to find out where people gather and what papers/magazines are most widely read. Use specific community papers and radio stations to get the message across. (See section below on **Making the most of the media**.)

It is important that your publicity makes clear that carers are needed for children according to their racial and cultural backgrounds. This will help to give communities the message that they are needed and valued. When advertising for specific children the issues outlined on page 10 regarding protection of the child's and family's identity will need to be considered.

Making the most of the media

The best publicity is often free publicity. The media (press, radio, TV) are desperate to fill space. But what stories do they want?

Read the local paper, watch or listen to the local news – you'll soon get the idea! The staple diet of local media is human interest stories – real stories about real people in situations with which readers, listeners and viewers can identify. Fortunately, Shared Care offers lots of opportunities for great human interest stories.

Step 1

- *Identify your story:* an event; anniversary; or carer's experience.

Step 2

- *Write a press release:* one side of A4, double spaced.
- Intriguing *headline;* spell out why it's a good story without going over the top. Make sure the salient points are in the first paragraph.
- Include *quote.*
- Give date, time, address and contact numbers for interview and photo opportunities.
- Additional information on separate page(s) giving details of your organisation and what you want to achieve through this press release.

Step 3

- *Contact media.*
- Phone to find out who to send your press release to: send it up to one week before the event.

Step 4

- Check two days before event; ring round; make sure people are coming.

Step 5

- *Follow up* on responses from public.
- Write to the media who turned up and thank them for their involvement or for featuring your scheme.
- Make contacts for the future.

Videos

The following videos are available; however, some may be rather old and the language and terminology used may not agree with current thinking.

Sharing the care, Northamptonshire Family Link Scheme. This 11-minute video can be used for recruitment of carers or for information for users and professionals. It shows an outline of what the scheme is about, including comments from carers, parents and children who use the scheme. Cost £25 (plus VAT). Contact: Social Services Department, Cottingham Road, Corby, Northamptonshire NN17 1TD;
Tel (01536) 401104.

Sharing the care, Shared Care Network, South East Group (1999). An introduction to shared care for parents and carers. Answering often-asked questions and telling their own stories about shared care. Cost £40 incl P&P. Duration 8½ minutes. Available from Action Video Services Ltd, 19 Glanmire, Billericay, Essex CM11 1DU;
Tel (0800) 389 8730.

Stockport Sharecare, 20 minutes. Gives an overview of scheme. Available on loan for £10 from Sharecare, Overdale Centre, Powick Drive, Romiley, Stockport SK6 3EF; Tel (0161) 494 5771.

The Shared Care Scheme, The Portland Project in Birmingham. A promotional video for both parents and carers giving an overview of a scheme. Approximately 16 minutes long. Available in English, Urdu, Punjabi, Gujarati, Bengali and Cantonese. Cost £60 + P&P from The Portland Project, 4 Dwellings Centre, Quinton Road West, Quinton, Birmingham B32 1RJ; Tel (0121) 303 5313.

Kent Family Link Scheme video depicts five children and five link families and explores all aspects of the Kent Link Scheme. 20 minutes long. Cost £25 + P&P, available from Kent Link Family Scheme, South Downs, Chequers Hill, Doddington, Sittingbourne, Kent ME9 0BN; Tel (01795) 886 242.

Access to services

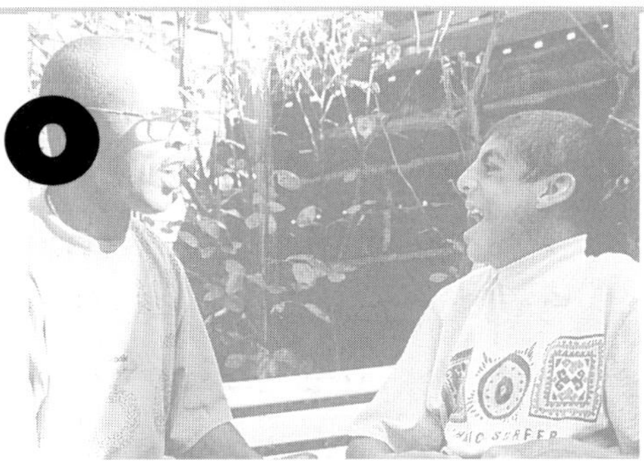

2

This section will explore ways of making services accessible to all sections of the community. Areas covered include:

- ideas for identifying local populations in order to assess whether the scheme is representative;
- if it is not representative, how groups who do not use the service can be targeted;
- access points – ideas are offered for a variety of outlets for publicity;
- ways of deciding who is eligible to use the service;
- monitoring and evaluation.

Legislation and guidance

The 1989 Children Act states that every local authority shall publish information about services provided by them under the following sections:

- *Section 17: the general provision of services to children in need*
- *Section 18: day care provision for children*
- *Section 20: the provision of accommodation*
- *Section 24: the provision of advice and assistance.*

The 1989 Children Act defines a category of children in need for whom the social services department should provide services. A child is defined as being in need if:

a) he/she is unlikely to achieve or maintain, or have the opportunity of achieving or maintaining a reasonable standard of health or development without the provision for him/her of services by a local authority under this part [of the Act];

b) his/her health or development is likely to be significantly impaired, or further impaired, without the provision for him/her of such services; or

c) he/she is disabled. (1989 Children Act Guidance and Regulations, Vol 6, Section 3.1)

Where they consider it appropriate, the local authority shall also publish information about services offered by others which the authority has power to provide.

In addition, the legislation states that local authorities should take such steps as are reasonably practicable to ensure that those who might benefit from services receive the information relevant to them.

Putting it into practice

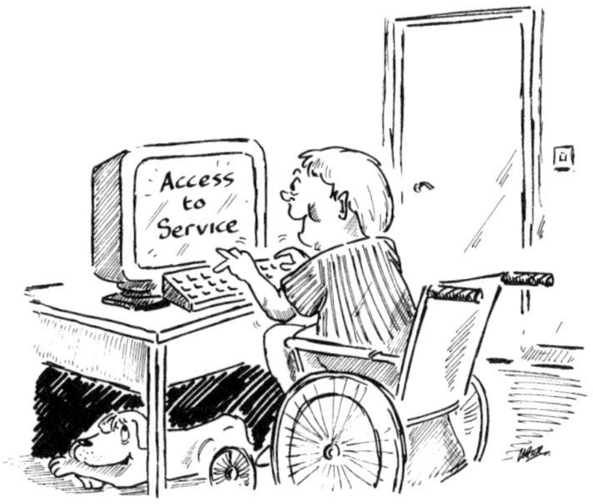

The local authority should ensure that their publicity material is in plain language and in large print. It should include a step-by-step guide which makes clear who may be eligible for the services provided and how they can make use of them. Publicity material should promote attractive, positive and non-stigmatising imagery, that is, images should fully reflect the make up of the community and show disabled children being active, not passive. The images should also reflect the age range of people who use the service and portray children and young people engaged in age-appropriate activities.

Information should be available in a variety of formats which can be understood by all sections of the community irrespective of age, ethnic origin, gender or ability. This should include media which take account of linguistic and cultural factors and the needs of people with communication or sensory difficulties.

At all times service provision, whatever the nature of the service, should be offered in a framework of anti-discriminatory practice and equal opportunities in the broadest sense.

If the local authority in your area is carrying out its obligations under the legislation, leaflets will have been translated into appropriate languages. If this is not the case, offer the authority some constructive advice, for example, present a list of local translators and costings or use the Shared Care Network leaflets which have been translated into six languages (see page 4 for details). The authority's information service or press and public relations department should have this information. Translators are also listed in Yellow Pages.

Advice can be offered on the content of leaflets and subsequent distribution to current users, special education networks and the local community health council.

Are you meeting the needs of your community?

What is the make up of the population in your area?

To find out contact the Information section of the local authority or consult the most recent Census material which is available in libraries. Another route would be via the Director of Public Health who has to produce an annual report. This will certainly include some demographic details relevant to determining potential local need.

Who is using your service?

Using the demographic data you can assess whether your scheme is representative. You may find that certain groups are significantly under-represented, eg families on low incomes, specific minority ethnic groups. This exercise will help you to formulate a publicity strategy and target specific areas or pockets within the authority where there is a low take-up.

Access through planning structures

Since the 1989 Children Act services have been increasingly required to look specifically at the needs of disabled children alongside non-disabled children and to ask the following key questions:

- Who are the children?
- What are their needs?
- What have we got currently or what do we need to develop, which addresses these needs in a way which is both effective and value for money?

Children's services plans

These are mandatory documents for local authorities which require joint planning with health, education and the voluntary sector. Within the document will be a chapter on children with disabilities which looks at current and changing need and service priorities. These documents are public and are updated annually.

Register of disabled children

A register is a requirement of the 1989 Children Act (Schedule 2).

Registers vary in quality and use, but good registers make a significant impact on real consultation and service development. A useful source of reference on this subject is *Positive partnership in developing registers of children with disabilities* (Preston and Russell, 1997).

Early years partnership

Changes in the structure of early year services, that is, for children aged 0-8, have led to the development of multiagency partnerships. These are responsible for producing an Early Years directory of services, reviewing current services and for formulating policy change and service development. They also review and develop policy and services.

Good inclusive policies at this stage mark the foundation of good inclusive services throughout a child's development.

The changing nature of disability and the changing demands on shared care services make these key structures for schemes to access and influence.

Access points

The scheme's publicity and information materials should be readily available from a network of sources such as local social services offices, health organisations, schools and play groups, benefit agency offices, council offices, a comprehensive list of voluntary agencies, shops and Post Offices as well as places of worship.

Health, education and social services departments are especially important agencies to target. Consider sending information to:

- special care baby units;
- social workers in children's divisions;
- portage workers;
- child development centres;
- community paediatricians;
- health visitors;
- physiotherapists, occupational therapists, speech therapists;
- educational and clinical psychologists;
- nursery education and day care services;
- paediatric departments in district general hospitals;
- special schools;
- GP surgeries.

Open days

Open days or evenings are a good opportunity for people to find out more about the service and to meet current carers, parents and users of the service. The following is an example of the publicity used by one scheme to encourage this.

Dear

Thank you for your interest in becoming a carer for *Families Together.* Enclosed is some basic information about the project. If having read it, you are still interested in working with us, we would suggest that you come to one of our open meetings. This will allow you to find out more about the sort of children we work with, what is involved in being a short-term carer and how our assessment process works. Our open meetings are held three times a year, usually in January, May and October, either in the morning from 10am–12noon or in the evening from 7pm–9pm. Anyone attending is expected to be here for the full 2 hours.

The next meetings are on the 19 and 24 January at the *Families Together* office. Please complete and return the enclosed reply slip in the envelope provided.

Yours sincerely

- -

Name: ....

Address: ....

I will attend the next opening meeting 10am–12noon — Yes/No

I will attend the next open meeting 7pm-9pm — Yes/No

I am not able to attend either meeting but am still interested in becoming a short-term carer — Yes/No

I am no longer interested in becoming a short term carer — Yes/No

Responding to enquiries

Responses from scheme coordinators or service providers should be prompt and courteous. People making an enquiry should receive a response within two weeks. This could take the form of either an acknowledgement card or a visit. At the point of enquiry the scheme worker may need to reiterate the eligibility criteria for children so that families are aware of the service's limitations. Some children may need to be referred to another service or agency.

Realistic feedback as to the likelihood of their child's needs being met within a reasonable time-scale should be given to parents. At an early stage, parents should also be informed of the procedures that will be followed before placement is arranged.

All communities have access points – they are just not all the same!

Your publicity strategy should include creative ways of getting your information to the groups you have identified as under-represented. *Some useful access points are:*

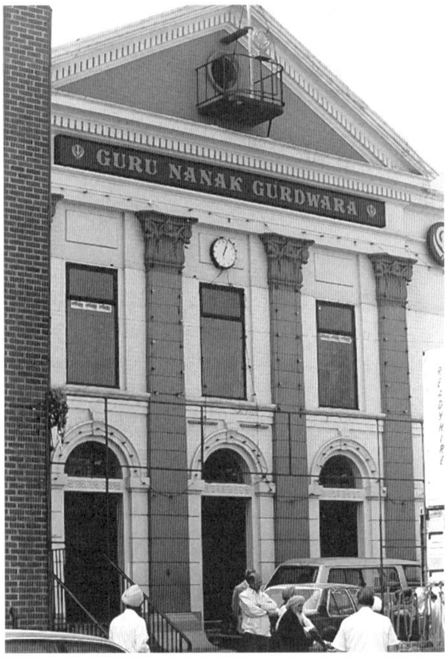

- key leaders in the community, rabbis, imams, church leaders

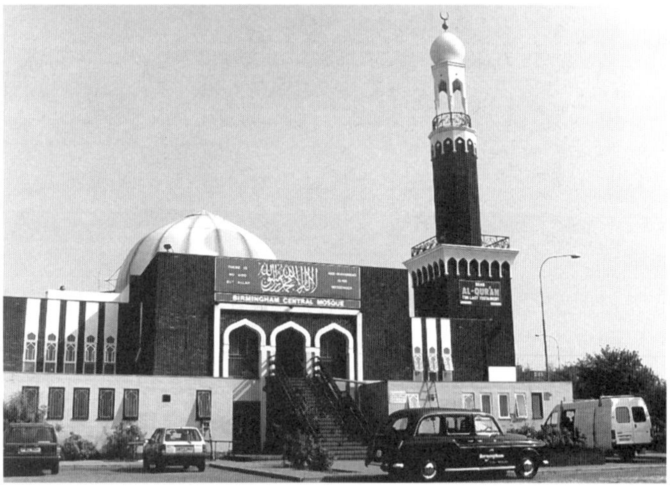

- key areas where communities gather, for example, target well-used community facilities which serve certain groups, libraries, GP's surgeries, Citizens' Advice Bureaux, community health councils

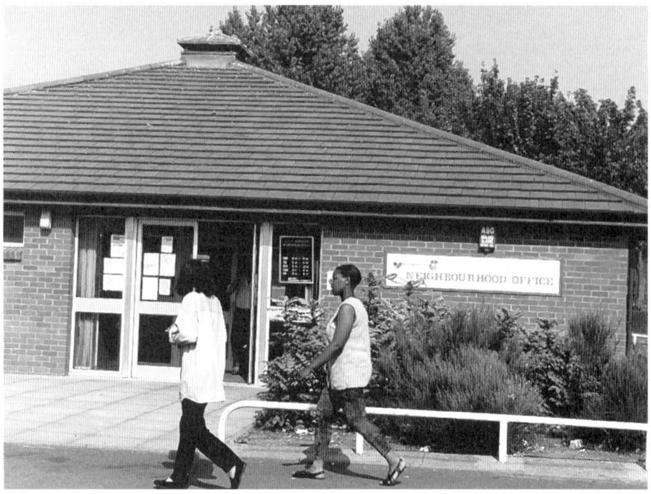

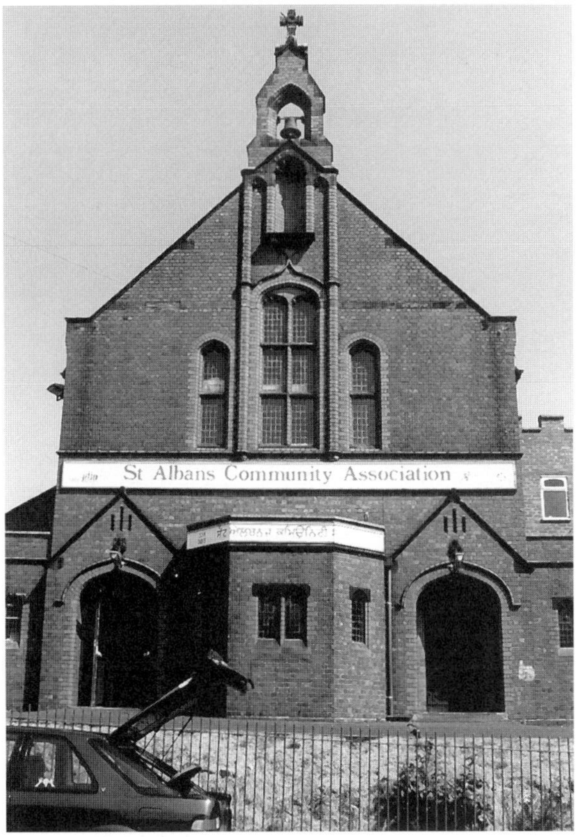

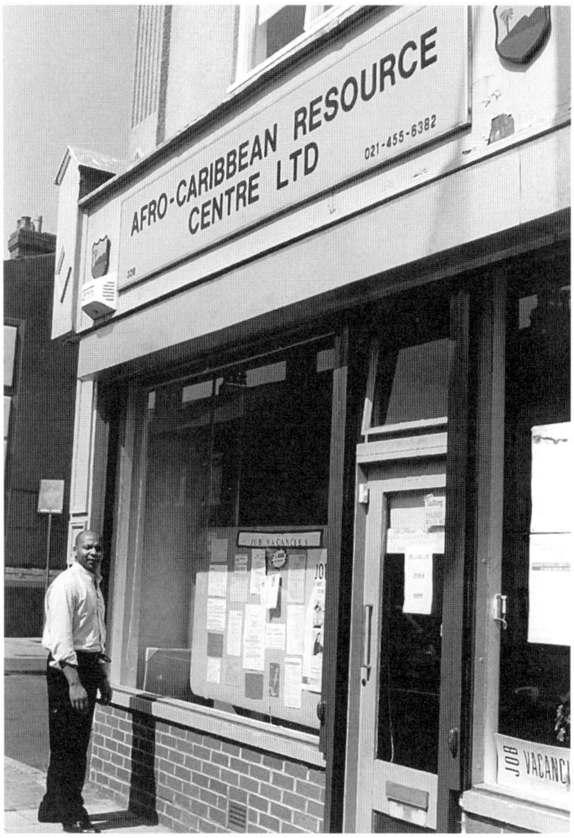

- voluntary agencies representing particular minority ethnic or other relevant groups, for example, disability groups, tenants groups, Contact a Family

Remember ...

Leaflets and posters distributed in the area should be in the appropriate languages.

Deciding on eligibility criteria

Government reports have consistently highlighted the need for all services to have clear, consistent and fair eligibility criteria (see SSI, 1994, 1998a, 1998b).

When deciding on criteria, services need to be clear about:

- whether a professional assessment or self-assessment is applicable;
- whether their own priorities match those of the social services department;
- whether criteria works inclusively and services do not exclude people;
- the method of recording whether unmet needs exist;
- whether the criteria reflects both the needs of the child and those of the family's circumstances.

Criteria for services needs to be communicated openly to current and prospective service users.

Monitoring accessibility

There should be a built-in monitoring process to assess whether all those who are eligible to do so are using the service. This should involve an annual review to assess numbers of new referrals and their breakdown, that is, geographical location, ethnic group, economic status, age and types of disability, date referred and dealt with.

To conclude, information about services should be made widely available to all sections of the community to enable them to make informed decisions about whether to use the services on offer.

Assessing carers

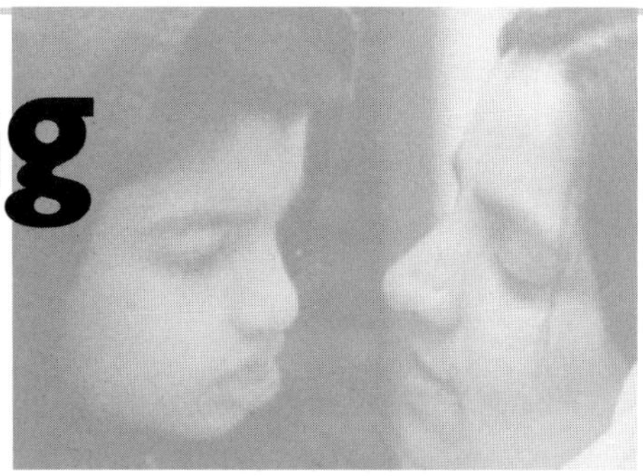

3

This section gives an overview of the considerations that need to be taken into account when assessing carers, and looks at:

- the reasons for assessing carers;
- when an assessment should take place and who should carry out the assessment;
- the process of assessment and the legal checks that need to be carried out;
- outcomes and terms of approval.

Legislation and guidance

Regulation 3 requires authorities to obtain information on and consider the range of factors set out in Schedule 1 in order to determine whether an applicant can be considered suitable to be a foster parent and whether his household is suitable for a child to be placed in....The aim should be to identify all the factors which contribute to a general picture of the applicants, their family and way of life.

Authorities and those interested in becoming foster parents must understand that an authority's duty is, unequivocally and unambiguously, to find and approve the most suitable foster parents for children who need family placement....

Fostering decisions must centre exclusively on the interests of the child. (1989 Children Act Guidance and Regulations, Vol 3, Sections 3.13-3.14)

Introduction

Assessment of carers is a two-way process. It allows the agency to obtain information on a carer's suitability to offer care to a child, and also gives carers an opportunity to explore the implications of providing short-term care in their family. Further reasons for carrying out assessments are given below and important factors that need to be considered are addressed throughout this section.

Why assess?

- The legislation requires it.
- It gives parents confidence in the service.
- It builds in safeguards.
- It gives carers time to explore options.
- The process allows carers to assess whether they have the space and time in their family lives to offer support.
- It helps the scheme make a judgement on a potential carer's suitability.
- The detailed information obtained is useful for subsequent matching.

A good assessment will allow carers to explore the implications of providing short-term care in their family.

Timing of assessment

There are a number of options.

The **first** is to assess before providing preparation. The advantage of this method is that you can be sure that the carer's skills, abilities and motivation are suitable. The disadvantage is that you do not get to know the carer in a wider setting, that is, interacting with other carers, discussing relevant issues.

The **second** option is to run assessment and preparation concurrently. The advantages of this method are that it reduces the total amount of time required to prepare and assess people and the process is more efficient. In addition the preparation may help applicants assess their own suitability and allow them to opt out. In the event of scheme workers deciding applicants are not suitable, they should be counselled out appropriately. This could involve sharing the reasons with applicants in a personal interview (apart from confidential third-party information) which is followed up in writing, and providing information on any appeal process available to them.

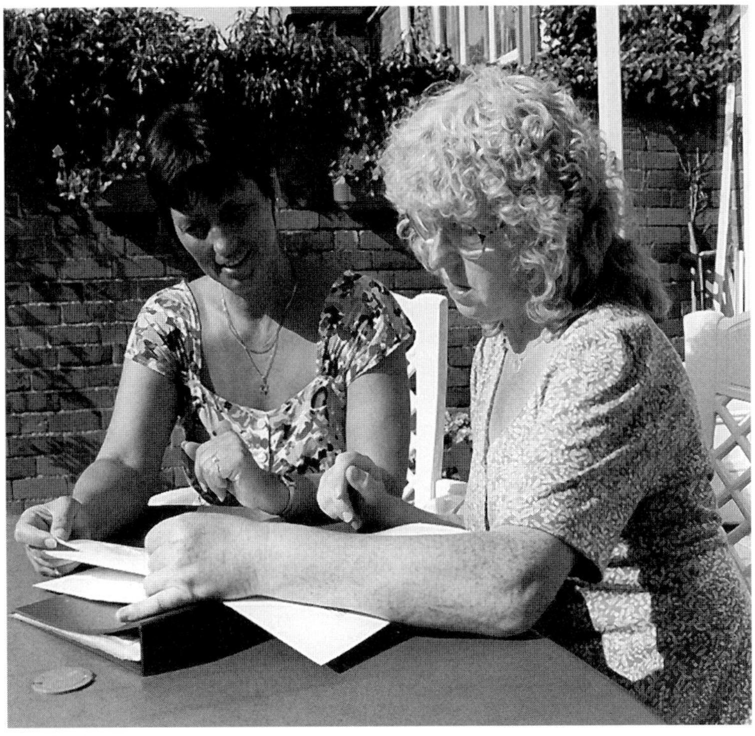

The disadvantages are that the role of assessor and preparer may become blurred and inhibit carers' contributions to the group.

The **third** option is to offer some preparatory sessions prior to assessment. While this method would mean that carers had a good idea of what is involved and would be committed, should carers prove unsuitable after preparation, this may be damaging to the carer's self-esteem and an inefficient use of resources.

It is clear that there are advantages and disadvantages attached to each method. You need a clear rationale about why you are choosing one rather than another.

Who should assess?

There is a legal requirement that the person assessing foster carers should be an authorised officer of the responsible authority. This is likely to be a social worker.

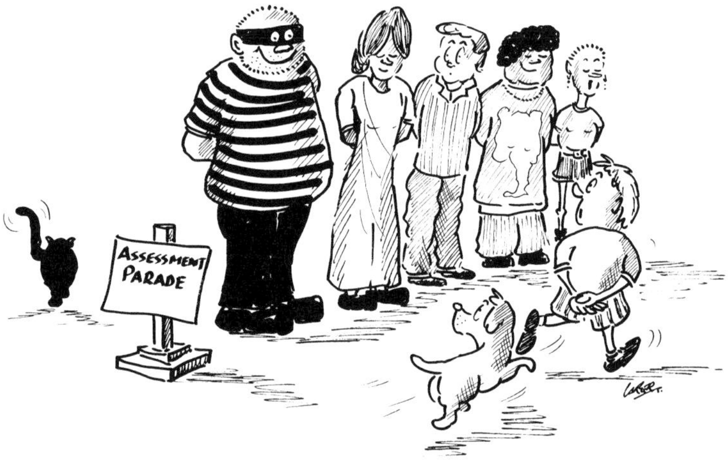

If anyone from a minority ethnic group is to be assessed then someone who is knowledgeable about their culture should be involved in the assessment. Special consideration may need to be given to providing interpreting services when the person being assessed and the assessor do not share the same language. This may mean spoken languages and sign languages.

The assessment process

Carers should be informed of the actual mechanics of the process prior to embarking on it. This information should include:

- why we assess;
- who assessors need to talk to;
- what sort of checks are made;
- how long it will take for the approval process to be completed;
- expectations made of carers during the process, for example, the number of preparation sessions they need to attend, approximate number of visits that the social worker will need to make;
- that the process will be treated as confidential to the agency;
- information on any policies the service has on smoking, pets, and so on;
- information regarding the service's expectations of carers, that is, minimum number of days they are expected to offer, number of compulsory training events, and so on.

During the assessment process, the following checks are legally required:

- ☑ police checks on all members of the household over 16 years of age or 10 years of age in Northern Ireland[1];
- ☑ full medical checks for the carers being assessed;
- ☑ social services department check;

- ☑ local regulations may require checks to be made with the education and housing departments of local authorities and with the probation service;
- ☑ interviews with two referees.

The process involves a number of document checks. These are:

- ☑ birth certificates;
- ☑ marriage certificates;
- ☑ naturalisation papers (where applicable);
- ☑ references – referees should be interviewed.

Carers should have an opportunity to comment on the report to be submitted for approval. Although it is not a legal requirement to have a panel, it is good practice for each responsible authority to do so. Although voluntary agencies are able to convene their own panels, panels must have a social services representative.

Each panel should either obtain a report from a medical advisor or have a medical advisor present. It would also be advantageous to have a social worker with experience of working with disabled children as well as carer and parent representatives on the panel. Panel meetings should be held at a time and place convenient to all members.

Shared Care Network has produced a booklet specifically for panel members (1997). *After careful consideration* contains information on the purpose and functions of a panel, roles and responsibilities and the differences between family-based short-term care and foster care. The booklet also contains case studies to help panel members consider a variety of issues that may arise.

Content

The British Agencies for Adoption and Fostering (BAAF) Form F is a useful tool for assessing carers, regardless of the amount of care they are providing. It is recognised, however, that some aspects of the form are not very relevant and require reduction while other sections require expansion.

The following are suggested as areas which should be explored further:

- an understanding of disability issues and expectations of disabled children;
- working in true partnership with children and families;
- race and racism;
- the carer's attitude to child-rearing practices, particularly with regard to discipline and vulnerability.

Carers could write the personal history section of the form themselves.

Shared Care Network is developing an alternative to the Form F specifically for family-based short-term care services. Copies of the forms will be available in 2000.

Note: If you keep personal information on computer you must register it under the Data Protection Act.

Outcomes

Terms of approval

These should be as specific as possible and cover the following:

- the number of children to be linked both at one time and in total;
- the age and ethnicity of the children;
- any relevant points concerning specific impairments or requirements to be met, for example, exclusions to children with certain disabilities because of the constraints of the accommodation.

Once approved, carers should receive a formal letter outlining the terms of approval and the foster care agreement.

Remember: Initial approval only lasts until the first annual carers' review. Account should then be taken of the skills and experience developed by carers.

Formal notification

Others who were involved in the approval process should also be given formal notification of the approval of the named carer. This is a legal requirement. (Arrangements for Placement of Children [General Regulations 1991] Regulation 5).

Note

[1] Amendment of the 1991 Foster Placement (Children) Regulations.

The amendment highlighted in a Local Authority Circular LAC (97) 17 relates to potential carers' criminal records. Prior to the amendment, social workers could exercise discretion regarding 'specified offences'. The amendment removes this discretion and requires that "responsible authorities shall not regard as suitable to act as a foster parent any person if he or any adult member of his household has been convicted of, or cautioned for, a specified offence".

These include situations where the conviction or caution was for an offence specified under Section 1 of the 1956 Sexual Offences Act (rape) or an offence specified in Schedule 1 to the 1933 Children and Young Persons Act.

However, in the case of some specific Schedule 1 offences, local authorities retain the discretion to consider the suitability of the foster carer.

Any approved carers or adult members of the household who have a relevant conviction or caution for a specified offence should have been reviewed following this amendment. Under the amendments "the existence of such a conviction or caution renders the person no longer suitable to act as a foster carer".

Assessing children and families

4

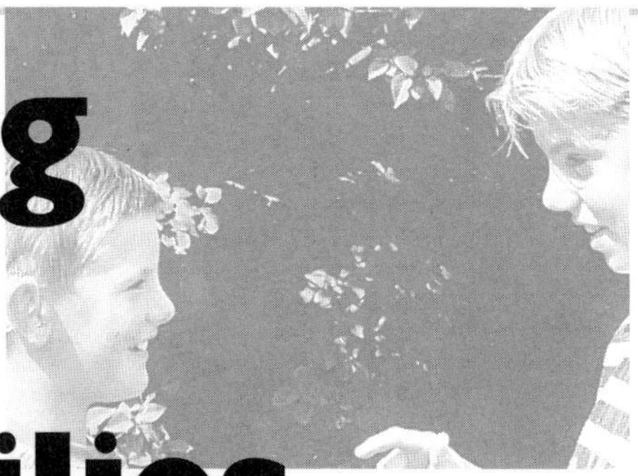

The focus of this section is on assessing the needs of children and families and the following questions will be addressed:

- Why assess?
- Who should assess?
- What should the assessment of the child cover?
- What should the assessment of the family cover?
- What should childcare plans contain?

Legislation and guidance

Social services departments need to develop clear assessment procedures for children in need within agreed criteria which take account of the child's and family's needs and preferences, racial and ethnic origins, their culture, religion and any special needs relating to the circumstances of individual families. (1989 Children Act Guidance and Regulations, Vol 6, Section 5.1)

The Act provides that a local authority may assess a child's needs for the purposes of the Children Act (1989) at the same time as any assessment under:

a) the 1970 Chronically Sick and Disabled Persons Act;

b) the 1981 Education Act (and now the 1993 Education Act);

c) the 1986 Disabled Persons (Services, Consultation and Representation) Act; or

d) any other enactment. (1989 Children Act Guidance and Regulations, Vol 3, Section 2.54)

The arrangements for Placement of Children Regulations place a statutory duty on responsible authorities to draw up a plan in writing for a child whom they are proposing to look after or accommodate in consultation with the child, his parents and other important individuals and agencies in the child's life (Regulation 3). Planning for the child should begin prior to placement. After placement, the plan should be scrutinised and adjusted (if necessary) at the first review ... and at subsequent reviews. (1989 Children Act Guidance and Regulations, Vol 3, Section 2.17)

Introduction

Assessment of children and families allows agencies to establish the needs of all parties for a short-term break. If family-based short-term care is the most appropriate service, the assessment will give the social worker full information regarding the child's strengths and needs and the families' expectations of the service. A recent Social Services Inspectorate report *Removing barriers for disabled children* (SSI, 1998a) reinforces the importance of coordinated joint assessments. The report highlights how families often feel frustrated at the number of parallel assessments that they are required to go through. Shared Care Network is supportive of key worker systems and where these systems are in place, scheme workers should refer to the key worker as a first point of contact. This section looks at the important factors that should be considered when assessing children and families.

Why assess?

- To look at the full range of the child's needs.
- To ensure that the provision of family-based short-term care is the most appropriate within the context of other options.
- To help families choose the most appropriate option for their child and family.
- To allow for the development of a proper childcare plan.

Timing of assessment and emergencies

The assessment process should be started before any consideration is given to accommodating a child. However, it is recognised that emergencies do occur and that a brief, rather than full assessment, may need to be carried out. This should always include basic information and a full assessment carried out at the earliest opportunity, ideally within 10 days. Where possible, arrangements should maintain and support attendance of the child's school or day care as these are significant stable factors in children's lives. If this is not possible, both are good sources of information about children, particularly on communication or on practical problems like feeding difficulties or management of equipment.

Basic information for emergency placements would include:

- the child's usual routine;
- details about health including medication;
- the child's doctor and emergency number;
- reason for placement;
- language, religion;
- details about the child's normal means of communication;
- education.

! *Note: In the event of a child being on a waiting list for more than six months there should be a reassessment of the child's and family's needs.*

Who should assess?

It is important that there is agreement between responsible agencies about who should assess the child and family. Whoever undertakes this role should ensure that all relevant parties have a copy of the assessment. If possible it is recommended that the child's social worker, and a scheme worker carry out a joint assessment. However, it is recognised that few children have a separate social worker and the task may fall to the link social worker.

The assessment process

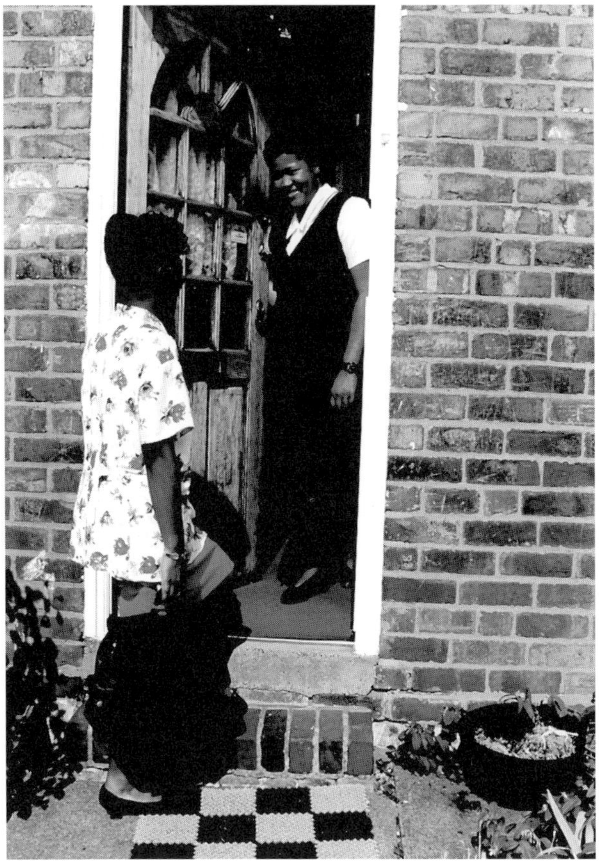

Most agencies will have an existing assessment form which can be used or adapted for family link purposes. Assessment should be carried out via home visits, school or day care visits, and interviews with families. It is important to observe the child in a variety of settings because a child who is described as having challenging behaviour at home may not present the same behaviour at school or vice versa. The child's view should also be sought directly (see parts of Section 6 on **Consulting children** for guidance).

What should the assessment of the child cover?

- health (see the end of this section for an example of a child health assessment form);
- disability;
- education;
- religious persuasion;
- ethnic origin;
- cultural and linguistic background;
- the degree (if any) to which these needs are being met by existing services to the family or child;
- which agencies' services are best suited to the child's needs.

Note: Families of children with special educational needs may benefit from having a named person as described in the Code of Practice associated with the 1993 Education Act. This person will have the task of supporting the family during and after assessments of special educational need. This person may be able to advocate for the family and practitioners will have to be receptive to working with this person.

Health requirements

Under the regulations a health assessment is still required before the placement begins, or as soon as practicable thereafter. The guidance suggests that information should be collected from the child's parents and, where appropriate, comments obtained from the child's GP about the child's health needs prior to placement. It is considered good practice to have information from parents about drugs and treatment programmes verified by the GP. The comments should be in written form. Any changes to medication or therapeutic treatments should be documented and passed on to carers, as should any forthcoming medical appointments. The following is an example of a letter.

Dear Doctor

1989 Children Act – 1995 Revisions to Regulations No 2015

Re:

The above child has been referred to us for placement with another family on a short-term care basis. Prior to the child's first stay with a link family, a medical examination and a health assessment are required. We have chosen to do this by consulting the parents and asking them to fill in a child health record which is enclosed. We would be grateful if you could:

a) verify the details on the record;

b) state whether the child has been examined in the previous three months either by yourself, the school doctor or the child development team.

In order to comply with the regulations can you please fill in the attached form and return it to us with the health record. I also enclose a consent form signed by the parents.

Please contact me if you wish to discuss this further or if you have any queries.

Thank you for your help with this.

Yours sincerely

Note: For children with complex healthcare needs a more detailed assessment will be necessary. Towards a healthy future (Servian et al, 1998) gives detailed guidance and examples of a range of forms.

What should the assessment of the family cover?

Assessment of families' needs should take account of:

- the family profile;
- their current support networks;
- the reasons for the request at this time;
- their experience of previous or other services;
- the family's expectations of the service.

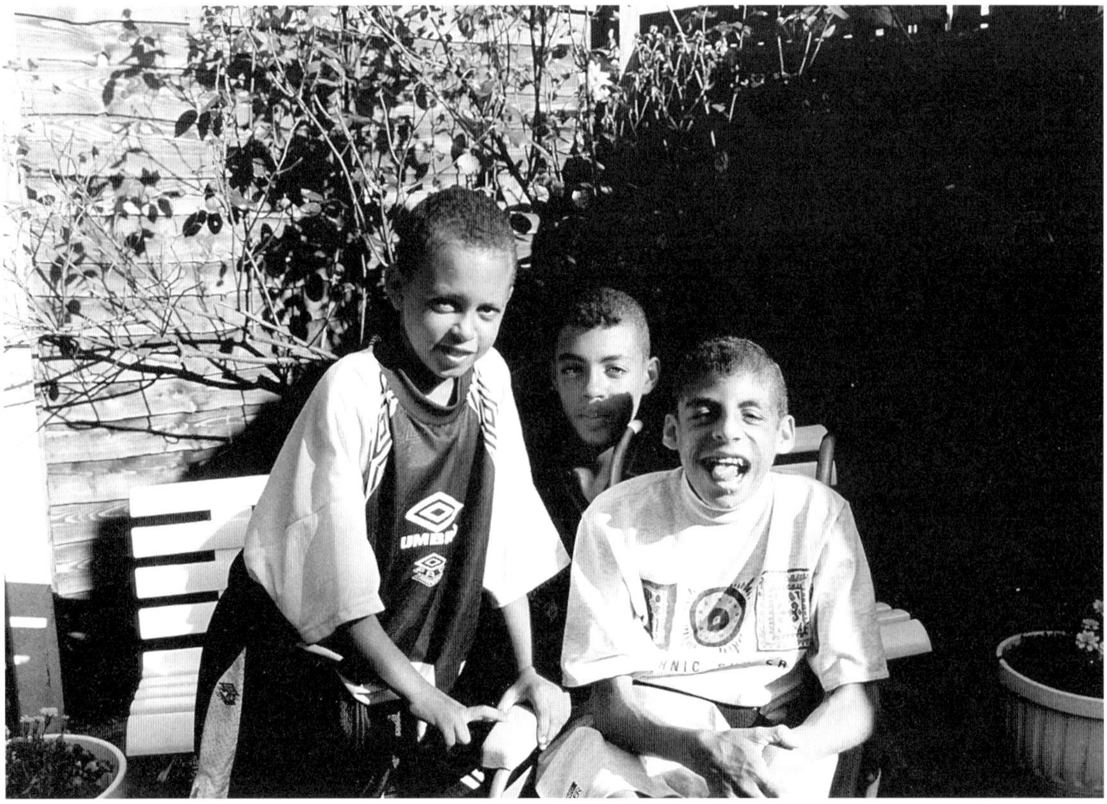

Families should receive a copy of their assessment which they may want to use to access other services. Following assessment the conclusion may be that family-based short-term care is not the most appropriate resource and a referral should be made to another service.

If, after the assessment is complete, it is deemed that shared care is the most suitable service, the social worker should be left with full information about the family's expectations of the service and their child's strengths and needs.

When carrying out assessments, people should be alert to the fact that there may be child protection concerns. It is important not to underestimate the extent of abuse towards children with disabilities and workers should use the established child protection procedures if they are concerned.

Once a full assessment has been completed a childcare plan should be drawn up.

Content of childcare plans

The plan should be recorded in writing and contain the following elements as described in the 1989 Children Act Guidance and Regulations, Vol 3:

- the child's identified needs, including needs arising from race, culture, religion or language, special educational or health needs;
- how those needs might be met;
- aim of plan and time-scale;
- proposed placement (type and details);

- other services to be provided to child and/or family either by the local authority or other agencies;
- arrangements for contact;
- support in the placement;
- likely duration of placement;
- contingency plan if placement breaks down;
- arrangements for ending the placement (if made under voluntary arrangements);
- who is responsible for implementing the plan (specific tasks and overall plan);
- specific details of the parents' role in arrangements;
- the extent to which the wishes and views of the child, the child's parents and anyone else with a sufficient interest in the child have been obtained and acted upon and the reasons supporting this or explanations of why wishes/views have been discounted;
- arrangements for input by parents, the child and others into the ongoing decision-making process;
- arrangements for notifying the responsible authority of disagreements or making representations;
- arrangements for healthcare (including consent to examination and treatment);
- arrangement for education;
- dates of reviews.

Looking after children

The 'Looking after children' materials were designed to improve the parenting experience of children looked after by local authorities. This was in response to research, which indicated that outcomes for children looked after by the local authority were considerably poorer than for children in the general population.

Shared Care Network recommends the use of 'Looked after children' forms with children with disabilities using family-based short-term care for less than 120 days or 90 days in Northern Ireland. For further information please refer to Shared Care Network *Children Act (1989) Policy group recommendations (1998)*.

The 'Looked after children' forms are not recommended to be used as a stand-alone comprehensive package in family-based short-term care schemes for children with disabilities. Rather, they need to be woven into the good practice that already exists within family-based short-term care schemes and which is outlined in *Stronger links*. The Department of Health plans to issue revised forms in 2000 that will be better tailored to disabled children and to short breaks.

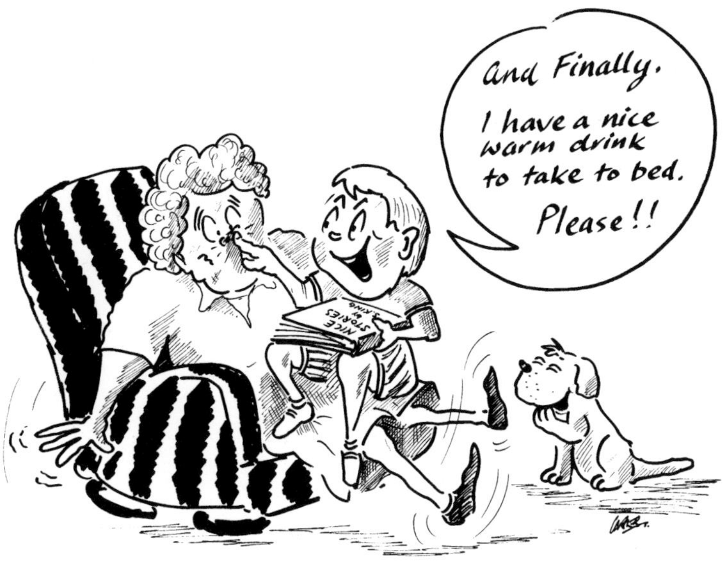

Profiles

As well as childcare plans there should be additional information provided to carers to ensure that they have full details about the likes, dislikes and normal routine of the child they will be caring for. An example of a profile used by a scheme is on the next page.

Additional information for carers/child profile

Child's name Address Tel no Date of birth	*Schooling* Does your child attend school,nursery or play group Yes/No If yes, which one Name Address Tel no Name of teacher
Child's GP Name Address Tel no	*Diet* Can you tell us what your child likes to eat and drink? Do they have any specific dislikes? Is there any food or drink they react badly to?
Emergency contacts Name Address Tel no Name Address Tel No	*Bedtime* Can you tell us your child's bedtime routine? What time does s/he go to bed? Do they have a particular pattern, for example, specific toys, light on/off, a hot drink?
Important people in child's life (please include brothers, sisters, pets, and so on) Is there anyone else involved with your child we would need to know, for example, parent advisor, health visitor? Please give details.	*Behaviour* In addition to child health record information is there anything else you feel the carer should know about your child's personality/ behaviour?
Details of child's special need **Important: For further detailed health and self-care information please read child health record which is attached.**	*Programme/routines* Can you tell us if there are any particular ways of handling your child that you or anyone else carry out, for example, school or portage? Are there procedures around toileting or eating or around handling any difficulties? What, particularly, might your child like in new situations?
Child's culture What language is spoken at home? Does your child speak any other language? Please give any details regarding your religion which would affect the care of your child (dress, diet, and so on).	Form completed on .... Form reviewed on .... Signed .... Designation ....

Child health assessment form

1989 Children Act

1991 Arrangements for Placement of Children (General) Regulations

Your child's name Address Tel no Date of birth	*Mobility* Please tell us how your child gets around. For example, can s/he walk, with or without help? Does s/he need to use any aid (for example, a buggy or a wheelchair)? Does s/he have any road sense?
Your child's doctor Address Tel no	*Teeth* Does your child have any problems with his/her teeth? Yes/No If yes, please give details.
Does your child have any specific medical problems? Yes/No If yes, please give details. Name of consultant and hospital	*Diet* Does your child have any special needs of problems with his/her eating? For example, does s/he require special food? Are there certain foods that should be avoided? Does food need to be presented a certain way?
Does your child have epileptic fits? Yes/No If yes, please give details (for example, how often, what warning signs are there, and is there a special way your child likes to be dealt with after a fit?).	*Allergies* Does your child have any allergies? Yes/No If yes, please give details.
Are your child's vaccinations up to date? Have there ever been any problems with vaccination? Has your child ever had an anti-tetanus injection? If so when?	*Behaviour* Is there anything about your child's behaviour you find difficult? Is there anything about your child's behaviour you think other people might find difficult? Yes/No If yes, please give details.

continued...

Does your child have any other medical problems, including sight or hearing difficulties? Yes/No

Does your child wear glasses or use a hearing aid? Yes/No

If yes to either of these questions, please give some details.

Medication

Is your child taking any medication? Yes/No

If yes, please give details.

Name of medicine/tablet/cream/etc:

Dosage:

When given and how:

Comment: It is important to list all medication, however often it is taken.

Toilet

Please tell us how your child attends to his/her toileting needs. Can s/he use the toilet unaided or does s/he need help? Does s/he use continence protection by day or night? If appropriate, is special help needed at certain times, for example, menstruation, constipation, etc?

Other health issues

If there is anything else you would like to tell us about your child's health or think we need to know, tell us here.

Please note: in addition to this written information please discuss all your child's needs with the short-term carer and the project.

Speech and communication

Does your child use speech to communicate? Yes/No

What language does your child normally use at home?

Does your child use any other form of communication, for example, sign language or BLISS? Yes/No

If so, what is it?

If your child has no formal communication methods, how does your child make his/her needs known to you? Please give details.

Does your child speak or understand any other language? Yes/No

If yes, please give details.

Completed by ....

....

In conjunction with ....

....

Relationship to child ....

....

Date ....

Reviewed on ....

Note: Additional forms for children with complex healthcare needs can be found in Towards a healthy future (Servian et al, 1998).

Preparation

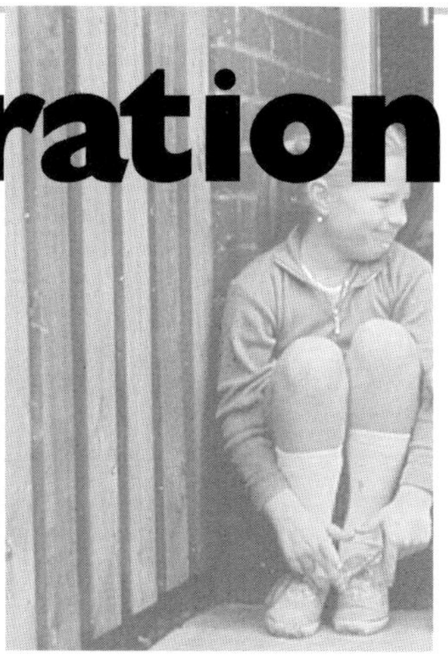

5

This section will look specifically at:

- the reasons for preparing short-term carers;
- core material which should be included in preparation sessions;
- what to include in a carer's pack;
- when and where group preparation sessions should take place;
- preparing families;
- what to include in a parent's pack;
- preparing children and young people for separation from home;
- preparing carer's children;
- the needs of siblings.

Legislation and guidance

Preparation should begin as part of the assessment process as the foster parent learns about foster care and what is required as foster parent. After approval, the social worker and foster parent should agree on what further preparation and training is needed before a child is placed and continuing beyond placement. (1989 Children Act Guidance and Regulations, Vol 3, Section 3.54)

Introduction

Preparation for a link is important, not only for prospective carers but also for families, the child or young person using the service and the carer's children. Issues around the preparation of all these groups will be considered in this section. At the end, the needs of siblings of children with disabilities are considered.

Preparing carers

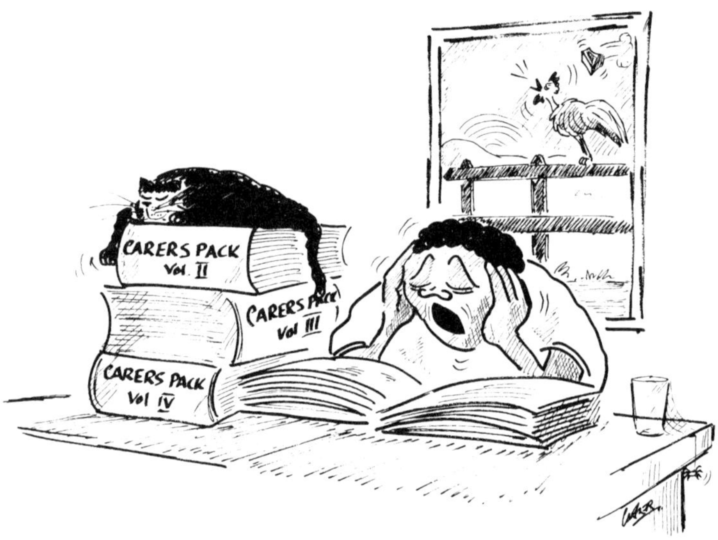

Preparation is the process which takes place between recruitment and training and may run in parallel with the assessment process. It is acknowledged that training should be provided throughout the career of a carer and attention given to their development. This will be covered in Section 10, **Training and support for carers**.

Why prepare short-term carers?

- It gives carers confidence and an enhanced sense of their worth.
- It helps assure both users and service providers that the quality of care on offer will be good.
- It gives carers a common knowledge base from which to continue learning.

- Carers can learn together and thereby form friendships and support networks.
- They can begin to understand the implications of short-term care for themselves and their families.
- It helps carers understand their relationship with the agency.

At the outset, it is important that potential carers are informed of the agency's preparation and training and made aware of the time commitment for the family or individual. Carers should be clear that the preparation sessions are mandatory. Preparation can take place in groups or on an individual basis. A combination of both approaches would be beneficial. Core material could be covered in group sessions whereas children's specific needs may require individual sessions, on issues such as feeding or lifting. If you are using group preparation sessions it is useful to enlist the help of an experienced carer to co-facilitate.

What core material should be included in preparation sessions?

In conjunction with the National Extension College, Shared Network produced a training manual called *When am I coming to stay?* This pack includes the components of a preparation course, which are considered to be important to cover:

- the effects of labelling and exploring participants' feelings about becoming a carer;
- working with the family of a child with a disability;
- considering the differing needs of children including the need to recognise and promote their cultural identity and how these needs may be met;

- the skills of caring and exploring carers' own values and how they may affect their work;
- the responsibilities of caring – confidentiality, policies and procedures for child protection, coping with challenging behaviour;
- a positive partnership – safety in the home, exploring carers' training needs, the rewards of caring.

A useful option is to take carers to the child's school or link up an existing carer and a potential carer for a day. It may also be helpful for carers to meet and talk with a parent who uses the scheme. A survey of carers' views about services (Newitt, 1997) indicated that many support carers are interested in becoming more involved in the scheme. This could include becoming involved in preparation and training sessions for new support carers and providing a mentoring system for people who are newly linked. This would not only draw on their useful skills and experience, but may also make carers feel valued. Carers' input into preparation should, of course, be appropriately recompensed.

Carers' packs

Carers' packs of information should be given out to carers at the beginning of the preparation and referred to throughout this period.

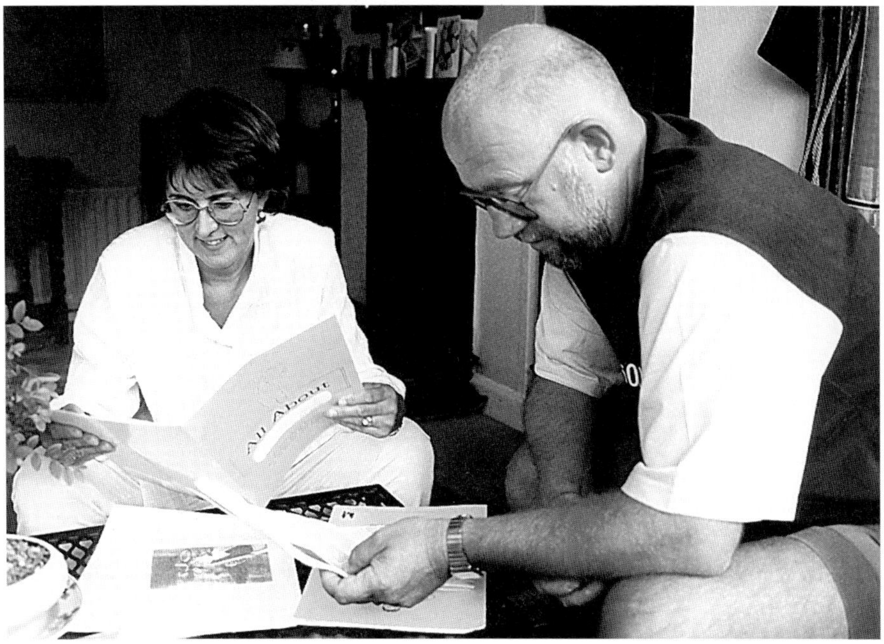

What to include in your carers' packs

Basic information on:

- child protection procedures;
- tax, insurance and benefits;
- approval and notification procedures including ongoing support available to carers;
- carer/child placement agreements;
- emergency procedures;
- comments, compliments and complaints procedures;
- the agency's policy on behaviour management and control;
- safety in the home;
- same-race policy;
- *Help starts here* – a pocket-sized reference book on sources of help and information (Council for Disabled Children, 1995);
- policies on complex healthcare.

Optional extras to include:

- guidance on intimate care;
- HIV/AIDS and infectious diseases;
- moving and handling;
- basic disability information;
- information on local voluntary agencies;
- useful addresses.

When and where should group preparation sessions take place?

Many carers have work or family commitments and their particular needs should be taken into account when scheduling sessions. Evening meetings are often the most convenient. You may also want to consider whether the sessions should be short and spread over a period of weeks or consolidated into two full days at the weekend. Consult carers to see which is preferable to the majority.

The choice of venue will depend on how many carers are being prepared. Make sure it is comfortable and accessible, with room for group exercises, that there are extra rooms if people need to split up into discussion groups, and that all of the necessary audio-visual equipment is available and working!

The venue needs to foster a relaxing atmosphere which will encourage group discussion. Comfortable chairs in a U-shape are more likely to put people at ease than hardback chairs around a boardroom table. Give consideration to providing a loose-leaf binder or wallet in which carers can keep their papers together.

Preparing families

Families who consider using shared care may feel apprehensive. Service providers should aim to help parents with these feelings. Ann Griffith, in *'When am I coming to stay?'*, suggests holding structured sessions for parents and involving a parent with experience of the scheme to co-facilitate.

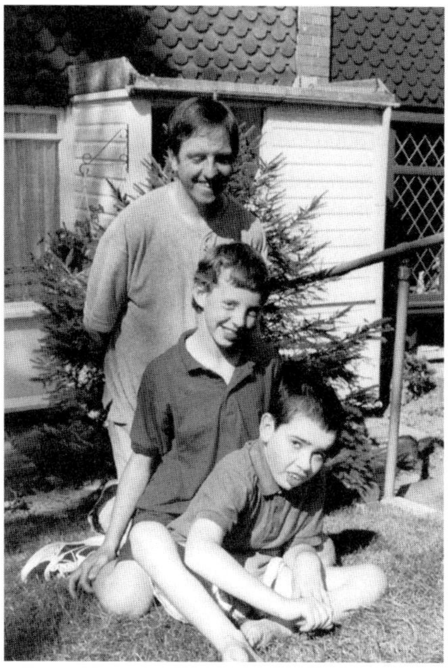

These sessions should:

- help parents think about what link care might mean for their child;
- help parents express any anxieties they may have about sharing the care of their child;
- work towards establishing a positive partnership between parents, carers and scheme workers in the care of the child;
- familiarise parents with the procedures of the scheme and the requirements of the 1989 Children Act.

Parents' packs

Issuing parents with a parents' pack would allow them to know what to expect from the scheme.

What to include in your parents' packs:

- written agreement (this is a legal requirement);
- list of relevant contacts;
- emergency phone numbers;
- their entitlement to the service;
- vouchers (if relevant);
- information about reviews;
- transport arrangements;
- what they can expect for their child;
- insurance information.

Preparing children and young people for separation from home

All children, regardless of their disability, should be prepared for using family-based short-term care services. When preparing a child for a period of separation from home the following points should be considered:

- early visits should take place in the child's own home;
- make introductory visits to carers short and ensure that the child is at first accompanied throughout the visit;
- provide photos of the link family with whom the child will stay;
- let the child dictate the pace of developments – unaccompanied visits should only be considered when the child is completely at ease with the carer;
- use methods of communication which the child can understand, for example, books which tell a story about leaving home to stay with friends and end with the person returning home, scrap books to keep a record of visits;
- make sure that the child has familiar toys or other favourite objects to take to the carer's home.

Who should prepare?

Children and young people should be prepared for separation by either the link worker or the child's social worker. Alternatively, there could be a combined effort with parents, teachers and relatives.

Options for preparing carers' children

Having a child to stay for short breaks involves the whole family and it is important that carers' children are not overlooked. They will benefit from good preparation too. Adapt the material given to carers for their own children and give carers pieces of homework which involve the whole family. At the end of preparation, invite children and established carers to a social event.

You may also want to consider working with carers' children in groups or on an individual basis. The following is an example of a preparation programme for carers' children used by Parents and Children Together (PACT), Yorkshire.

PACT Preparation Programme for Carers' Children

Introduction

- Welcome, location of toilets, parents, etc
- Name games

Looking at ourselves and others

Sit in a circle, throwing a bean bag to decide turns.

- Describe ourselves, other people in the group, our similarities/differences, likes/dislikes, what we are good at/or not so good at.

Look at pictures of children, positive pictures of children with and without disabilities in a variety of settings.

- Ask children to describe the picture: what activities are taking place? what other activities might the children in pictures enjoy, or find difficult?

Awareness of disability

The children take part in an activity that requires some dexterity, for example, drawing or doing a jigsaw. Then the activity is made more difficult by asking the child to use only the weaker hand or wearing a heavy mitt.

- Talk about feelings, difficulties, and frustrations; how might other people view their work.

Communication

Miming, learn some Makaton signs, then a nursery rhyme in Makaton (use the Makaton nursery rhyme video).

- Talk about the different methods of communication; why some children might need them. How do you feel when someone can't understand you?

Refreshments

Learn Makaton signs for different foods. Practice feeding each other (usually the group leader is the guinea pig!). Have refreshments!

- How might a child feel if s/he needs help with feeding? Introduce the idea that some children may need help with their personal care needs. Importance of dignity.

Sharing

Use worksheets – draw or make your house, with boxes for things to share or not to share.

- It can be fun to share; what would we share? It's OK not to share everything. What happens if something breaks?
- Sharing parents' attention.

The sessions are meant to be fun. If a child wishes to opt out of an activity, or take part in his/her own way, that's fine. Each child must have opportunities to speak in the group or individually while they are taking part in an activity about their feelings. Therefore, have a good ratio of adults (parents, carers, and scheme workers).

Sessions usually last two hours. They are best held in a child-friendly environment.

The needs of siblings

Many services are realising that the siblings of children with disabilities often feel excluded and to redress the balance are setting up siblings groups. The groups allow children to share their feelings about their brother or sister with others and gain support and understanding from their peers. Gill Priestley from the Bradford Family Placement scheme outlines some of the issues.

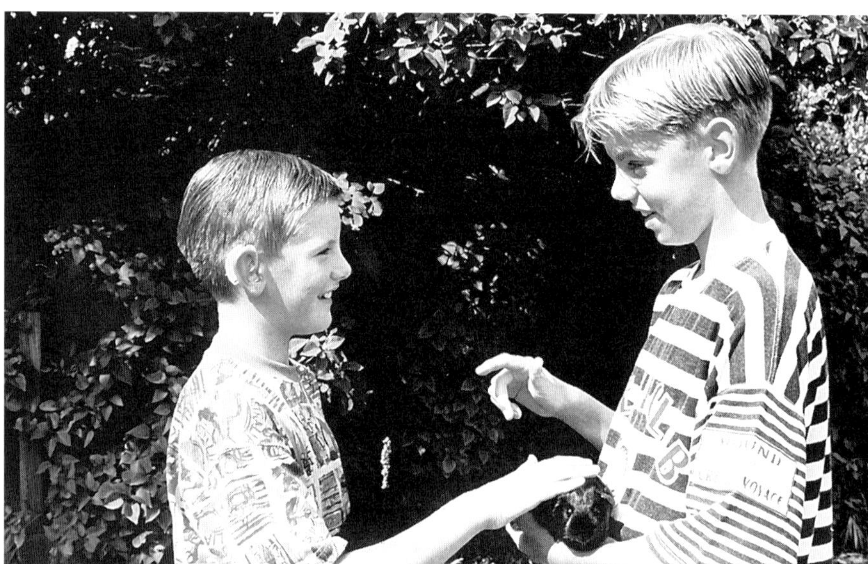

Concerns siblings may have include:

- worry about whether their brother or sister is safe;
- anxiety about whether they will return;
- jealousy – a feeling of 'missing out' or being 'second best';
- frustration at not being able to express their feelings due to sense of family loyalty.

Helping strategies for siblings

Some of the concerns mentioned above could be addressed by:

- providing information to ensure that they know where their sibling is staying;
- allowing children daytime visits at their sibling's support carer's home;
- holding social events which bring families together;
- running siblings' support groups.

Siblings' support groups

When setting up a siblings' support group, workers need to identify the aims and objectives of the group. These may include:

- giving the group members time and space away from their families;
- providing fun activities and a positive experience;
- allowing people to express and discuss their feelings about their family situations in a safe environment.

When organising a group, bear in mind the following factors:

- the choice of venue should be welcoming and suited to children;
- the timing of group sessions should be convenient to both the children and their parents;
- the length and number of sessions (sessions should not be too long otherwise some children may become overtired);
- the suitability of potential group leaders;
- the size of group and selection of its group members in terms of age.

The number of schemes running siblings' groups are growing. The groups offer children a safe environment in which to express their feelings and many children report very positive effects. The needs of siblings are an important aspect of family-based short-term care and should not be overlooked.

This section has offered suggestions for preparing disabled children, their siblings and parents in addition to link carers and their children. It is clear that good preparation is important for all concerned and an essential part of the linking process.

6 Consulting children, parents and carers

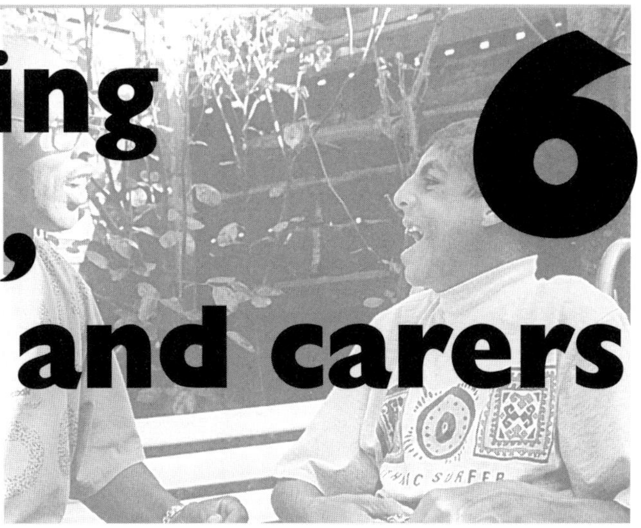

This section focuses on ways of consulting parents, carers and children about family-based short-term care services. It looks specifically at:

- reasons for consulting parents and carers;
- levels of partnership;
- reasons for consulting children;
- when to consult children and methods of doing so;
- issues to be aware of when consulting children;
- consulting children with few communication skills;
- advocacy;
- making consultation culturally sensitive.

Legislation and guidelines

One of the key principles of the Children Act (1989) is that responsible authorities should work in partnership with the parents of a child who is being looked after and also with the child himself, where he is of sufficient understanding, provided that this approach will not jeopardise his welfare.

A second closely related principle is that parents and children should participate actively in the decision-making process. (1989 Children Act Guidance and Regulations, Vol 3, Section 2.10)

The 1989 Children Act states that:

... before making any decision with respect to a child whom they are looking after or proposing to look after, a local authority shall so far is reasonably practicable, ascertain the wishes of, the child, his parents, any person who is not a parent but who has parental responsibility for him, any other person whose wishes and feelings the authority consider to be relevant regarding the matter to be decided. (1989 Children Act Guidance and Regulations, Vol 3, Section 2.46)

Introduction

In recent years there has been a recognition that obtaining the views of those who use services is an important element of good quality service provision. Indeed, the principle of consultation is enshrined in law. However, it is not always easy to do this effectively – especially if some of the people concerned are fearful about losing a service if they are in any way critical of it. Similarly, if people are not accustomed to being asked their opinions or have difficulty expressing themselves, creative approaches will need to be developed. This section attempts to look at the reasons for consulting and to identify ways of doing so effectively.

Why consult parents and carers?

In a telephone survey of parents' views of services (Newitt et al, 1997), 47% of the parents interviewed said that they would like to be more involved in the running of the service.

Parents should be consulted for a number of reasons. Firstly, to ensure that their needs are being met; secondly, to ensure that the service accommodates individual needs;

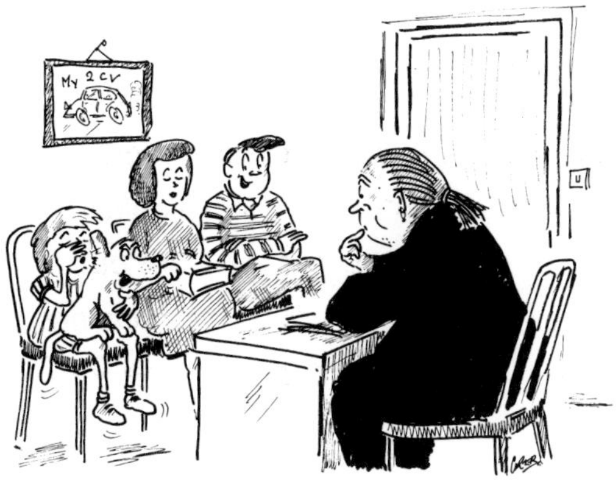

and thirdly, to enhance the partnership between parents and workers.

Carers should be consulted for similar reasons, as well as the following:

- to recognise that the service values them as an essential resource;
- to recognise that the service is accountable for their actions;
- to enable carers to deliver the best possible care;
- to ascertain training and support needs;
- to help promote the service – parents and carers may have helpful insights and ideas for the development of the service.

Levels of partnership

While partnership must be the goal we aim for, it is important to recognise that there are different levels of partnership. Pugh et al (1987) outline five different levels of parental involvement which are described below.

1 Non-participation

This may either be through choice because parents and carers have other commitments or due to other factors. For example, parents and carers may like to be involved but do not have the access/confidence or the right language skills.

2 Being there

Parents/carers may feel happy to come in and out of the scheme and stop for coffee and a chat. While they may make their presence felt they are not actively involved.

3 Cooperation

This means helping out with activities such as fundraising. However, the agenda for action is determined by the professionals not the carers or parents.

4 Collaboration

This occurs when carers/parents positively work with the scheme, for example, by helping to set up a new recruitment initiative, or a new support group, or working with other families and sharing their experiences of being part of the scheme. The parents and carers may work jointly with professionals on a particular project, but the professionals have the ultimate responsibility.

5 Partnership

There have been a number of attempts to define partnership in the social welfare field. Here are two that are frequently quoted.

> *A working relationship that is characterised by a shared sense of purpose, mutual respect and a willingness to negotiate. This implies a sharing of information, responsibility, skills, decision making and accountability. (Pugh et al, 1987)*

> *The basic principle, I believe behind a true partnership is sharing. A sharing of knowledge, of power, of resources, of information, of expertise and decision making. Partners are different but equal. (De'Ath, 1982)*

Both of these definitions emphasise the importance of sharing. In terms of family-based short-term care schemes this may mean:

- Partnership between individual carers/parents and schemes, for example, carers as co-workers or educators; carers sharing in reviews and assessments; parents as partners in an evaluating process or setting standards of quality.

- Partnership between carers/parents in general and with scheme workers, for example, this might mean:
  - participation in planning processes;
  - sharing in the formulation of aims and objectives;
  - sharing in finding particular carers for 'hard to place' children;
  - ensuring the representation of different community groups in the service.

- Carers and parents in partnership on policy – members of advisory or management groups or approval panels where their opinions are listened to and respected.

The important thing is to be clear where the service is on the scale. The dynamics of any service mean that it is likely to be at a different point on the scale with parents than carers. Services may also have reached a stage where the current level of partnership needs to be maintained. If so it is important to recognise this and be clear about why this level of partnership is appropriate.

Check

- Where is your scheme on the scale outlined above?
- Where would your parents/carers and children think you were on this scale?
- Where do you think the following example comes on the scale?

An example of partnership

Coordinator, Maureen Rice, explains how the Nottinghamshire scheme put partnership with parents and carers into practice.

In response to the 1989 Children Act the Home from Home coordinators in Nottinghamshire wanted to develop new publicity material – posters, leaflets and a video – which would provide information for parents and also be used for the recruitment of short-term carers.

It was agreed that it would be helpful to consult with people already directly involved in using and providing short-term care services so parents and carers were invited to an informal evening meeting. The task was to consider what messages would be appropriate when describing the needs of disabled children and what information was relevant for potential carers.

There was much helpful discussion and a consensus that information about disabled children should be positive and reflect their individual personalities. It was decided that there should be space for the children to speak for themselves and, as a result, there is a page on the leaflet for 'What the children say' and some children's drawings.

One of the major benefits of the evening was the opportunity for parents and carers to share ideas and, in being consulted, they knew that they and their children were actively influencing the publicity material for Nottinghamshire's Home from Home scheme.

Consulting children

Why consult children?

- It is a means of empowering children who otherwise have little control over their lives.
- It enables children to have a voice about the sort of care they receive.
- It is a measure of how sensitive your service is to the needs of the children using it.
- Children can give positive direction to the way services develop.
- It is a legislative duty under the 1989 Children Act.

When to consult children

- Children should be consulted during the assessment process – part way through the introductory period and before any commitment is made.
- Before the child stays overnight.
- Before reviews.

As outlined above, the 1989 Children Act requires service providers to consult the children who use their services. It is important that within a local authority or agency there is clear agreement about who is responsible for consulting specific children. The challenge is for service providers to find creative ways of allowing the child to express their views. One way forward may be to designate an officer to guarantee the children are included in the review process. This may be the reviewing officer for the authority or a worker who has special skills in a range of communication techniques.

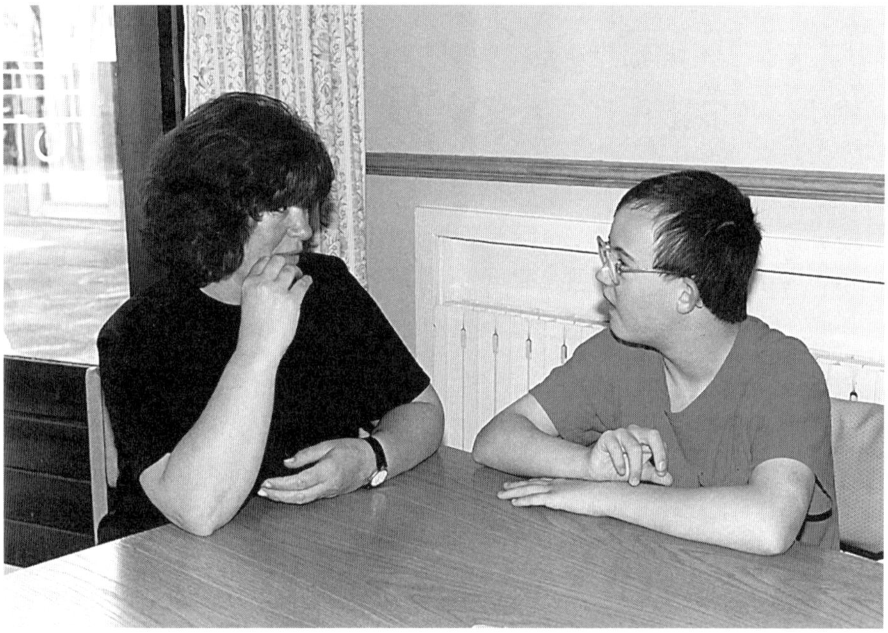

Issues to be aware of when consulting children

Sensitivity to parents' views

A particular issue which may arise when consulting children is that of actually discussing the child's disability. Some parents feel very strongly that they do not want their child to discuss this issue. However, this is unlikely to be avoidable in a family link situation and parents should be made aware of this.

Many services are now consulting children individually and in small groups about the services they receive. Some schemes have set up ongoing consultancy and advisory groups.

PACT Yorkshire describe a forum they use for consulting children.

'Take 10' is a young people's consultation and reference group. It is a forum where 10 teenagers, who have, have had, or hope to have a PACT link, can have their say about PACT family-based short-term care and future developments. The group meets six times a year for a mixture of working meetings and social activities. Working meetings are held in informal settings, usually a quiet corner of a leisure centre snack bar; social activities are chosen by the group themselves.

The group has developed its own sense of identity, deciding on its name, the venues where it will meet, which items it will discuss and the length of meetings. New members are invited onto the group by scheme staff in consultation with the young people, taking into account age, the gender balance of the group, commitment and the ability to contribute.

Scheme workers facilitate the meetings and enable those members with communication difficulties to be able to air their views. Much use is made within the group of video, tape recordings and visual prompts. The scheme workers then take the group's comments to the adult Advisory Group and ensure that the young people's views are heard when developing new pieces of work.

The group has contributed in the development of a new format for the family form to make it a more child-centred profile. They have also influenced the content of materials to prepare children for separation from their own family and for links with a new family. They have also contributed to a publication, *The way it is*, talking about issues which affect them in their everyday lives, and are currently working on a magazine article.

It has been important from the outset that the young people enjoy coming to the group, that it is organised in a 'teen-friendly manner' and that the young people feel free to speak out. Scheme workers try to keep in the background, though a balance has to be kept between adult involvement and the care, safety and communication needs of some members of the group.

As the vital importance of consulting disabled children has been recognised, there are a growing number of guidelines/ research reports available. Key references include:

Alderson, P. (1995) *Listening to children: Children, ethics and social research*, Barkingside: Barnardo's.

Morris, J. (1998) *Don't leave us out*, York: Joseph Rowntree Foundation.

Ward, L. (1997) *Seen and heard: Involving disabled children and young people in research and development projects*, York: Joseph Rowntree Foundation.

The Children's Society's *'I'll go first'* pack is a tool kit specifically developed for use in planning meetings and reviews with disabled children. It provides a set of boards with key questions on a range of care solutions, including family-based short-term care. Rebus and Makaton translations, pictures and stickers are designed to enable children to communicate their wishes and feelings. The Good Practice Guide in the pack suggests many ways of adapting the materials to suit children with differing means of communication. The boards are designed to enable both the child and the social worker to have a record of their views to take to a review meeting. For more information ring (0171) 841 4000.

Shared Care Network's own research (Prewett, 1999) which asked over 40 children and adults about their short breaks drew on work by Robinson et al (1996), Minkes et al (1994) and Morris (1998). These studies suggest that interview schedules should be devised in a concrete, logical manner relevant to the children's level of understanding. Pictures, symbols, signs, drawings, photographs of the child's family and link carers can be used to support the discussion and to record the individual's responses in a concrete form. Also, the use of sounds and smell can remind the child of places and events, while emotional faces (happy/sad) often allow children with little verbal communication to express their emotions.

Putting it into practice

Children with few communication skills

Observational techniques can be used to assess if children are happy. During the assessment process it is important to build up profiles of children, to ascertain how they express their feelings and to understand what certain behaviours indicate.

If it is not possible to consult a child verbally, it may be useful to develop a communication picture. Their parents will be very familiar with subtle behaviours and will be able to interpret them in terms of their emotional welfare. It is important to keep this information in written form so that it is available for reference when consulting children about the service.

The following suggests a method for consulting children with learning difficulties, based on the research by Robinson et al (1996) and Prewett (1999):

1. Always get parents' consent to the consultation exercise. Ensure that the child understands what is happening and gain their consent. Let them know they can stop if they want to.
2. The 'interviews' should be conducted by someone the child knows well but who will not try to influence the child's answers.

3. Use photographs of relevant people and places to help focus the child's attention on the service being discussed.
4. Use pictures of everyday objects such as food, games and places, for example, a park, to allow the child, with the interviewer's support, to build up a pictorial record. The researchers in the study mentioned above had stickers made depicting activities which children reported doing when away from home.
5. The interviewer should ask simple direct questions and record the child's response (verbal or non-verbal). The interviewer should be careful not to use double negatives.
6. Encourage interviewers to communicate with the child in whatever way is normal for them.
7. Try to avoid complex concepts such as same and different and the use of references to time. It is better to focus on specific events which take place near to TV programmes or meals.
8. Ask a mix of Yes/No questions and questions that allow children to give fuller answers, for example, 'Do you enjoy going to...?', plus, 'What do you like best about it?' Ask the question in a different way to ensure that they have understood. Don't be afraid to use 'jargon' they understand.
9. Try the questions out with a small group of children. Be prepared to change the wording if children cannot understand.
10. Don't despair – consultation takes time and practice. It is, however, a worthwhile exercise and as you become more experienced it will become easier (Robinson et al, 1996).

A communication picture for Accas

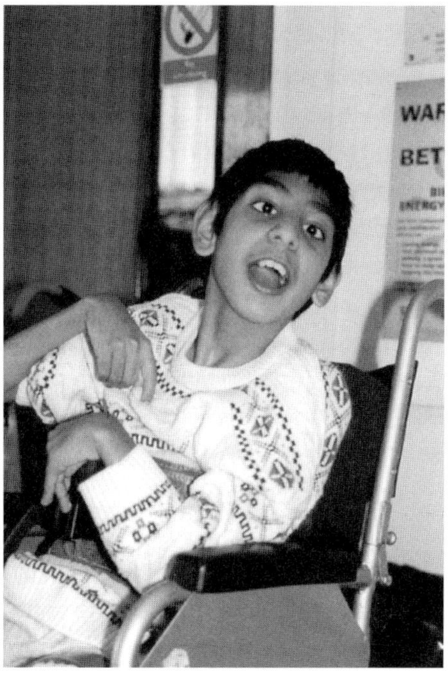

Accas is 12 – he has profound Cerebral Palsy. He has very restricted sight and no formal communication skills. He is, however, very able to make his needs known and uses his other senses well. He responds well to the sounds of voices he likes and deliberately turns away from sounds he dislikes.

Although he cannot actively play, he loves soft things, toys and scarves being placed on his face so that he can throw them away with his hand. When he is happy he will giggle and laugh, when he is not happy he will greet you with a silent glare.

Accas has a strong sense of smell and will deliberately clamp his teeth shut when food or medicine he doesn't like is aimed his way. When his favourite food, currently Rice Krispies, is offered he takes it easily and happily.

Accas can clearly show happiness and distress. When he is sad or uncertain he will cry and deliberately try to bang his head when he is happy he will smile and 'shout' at others.

All children, whatever their level of disability, can have communication plans like this. Such a plan helps with an assessment of a placement. It may be worth working with parents on compiling one for their child.

Using this information, innovative methods could be employed. For example, one could monitor the child's response to the sound of the carer's voice.

Advocacy

Citizen advocacy has been defined as "the development of a supportive, one-to-one relationship between an unpaid private citizen and someone who is vulnerable or at risk of isolation, with the aim of offering some protection to the latter and to help achieve his or her personal goals" (Simons, 1993).

In the context of family-based short-term care services an advocate may help the child express their views about their satisfaction with the short-term placement and highlight any changes they may want. Citizen advocacy is not just for children who have limited or no speech. It is also appropriate for people who are more able. If children do not have someone who acts as their advocate, you may be able to find someone appropriate to do so. Alternatively, you could access citizen advocacy organisations such as the Advocacy Alliances.

Self-advocacy is defined as "the process of individual development through which adults with learning difficulties acquire the skill and confidence to assert their own views" (Simons, 1993).

However, self-advocacy usually refers to groups of people with learning difficulties coming together to voice their concerns. It is possible that older children may have access to self-advocacy groups at school and these could be used effectively to discuss satisfaction with the services they receive.

Making consultation culturally sensitive

Consultation with parents, carers and children needs to be culturally appropriate. Culture influences services significantly – workers may have very particular white Western views on:

- family structures and life-styles;
- codes of conduct;
- child-rearing practices;
- employment or work.

White Western workers often walk into assessments of carers holding subconscious views on arranged marriages, the role of women, an approach to child-rearing and so on. One option could be to carry out the assessment with someone from the same cultural background who also understands the legal requirements. Another option would be to take the discussion back to the team to prevent one person's prejudice influencing the outcome.

Children, particularly those with more profound disabilities, often rely heavily on their five basic senses. We need to remember how much these respond to cultural cues.

Consultation should be with:

- someone who is well known to the child;
- someone who speaks the same language as the child/carer/parent;
- someone who is willing to use creative ways of communicating.

Remember to take into account important religious dates and festivals when choosing times for consultation and to adapt the materials for use with the children to ensure they are culturally relevant.

In summary, the views of parents, carers and children should be sought. The challenge for workers is to create an environment in which people feel able to express their opinions and to find creative ways of consulting children with few communication skills. Obtaining the views and opinions of the major stakeholders in the service is a vital element of good quality service provision.

Matching and linking 7

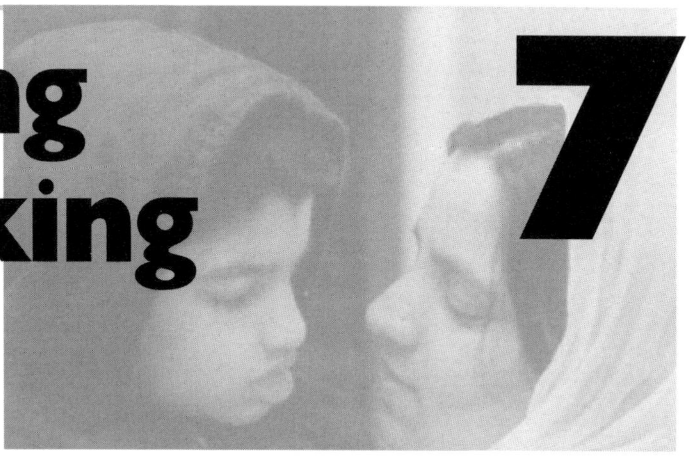

The aim of this section is to identify some of the important criteria that workers need to consider when matching children to support families. These include:

- ethnic origin;
- life-style;
- religion;
- the carer's environment;
- the carer's experience;
- the number of links per carer;
- written agreements.

The number of children a carer should be linked with is discussed and an example of a written placement agreement form is offered.

Legislation and guidance

A child's need for continuity in life and care should be a constant factor in choice of placement. In most cases this suggests a need for a placement with a family of the same race, religion and culture in a neighbourhood within reach of family, school or day nursery, church, friends and leisure activities. Continuity also requires placement in a foster home which a child can find familiar and sympathetic and not remote from his own experience in social background, attitudes and expectations. (1989 Children Act Guidance and Regulations, Vol 3, Section 4.4)

Introduction

Family-based care depends on those using the service and the carers who provide it having a positive relationship. This should not happen by chance: workers should have clear criteria for matching carers to particular children and families. This section considers which factors need to be taken into account when creating links and offers some practical examples of the kind of agreements that can be drawn up between carers and parents.

Once carers are approved and children assessed there should be clear information about the skills of individual carers, for whom they are willing to offer care, and how often they will do so. Good matching occurs when the child's and family's needs match what the carer has to offer.

Written or drawn profiles should be developed for the child and his/her family as well as the carer and their family. Examples of a form used to assess the child's needs can be found at the end of this section (**Matching detail form**). Also see Section 4 of the guide for an example of a **Child profile form**. If a child has complex healthcare needs a more detailed process needs to be conducted. For further details see *Towards a healthy future* (Servian et al, 1998).

The following factors need to be taken into consideration when matching families.

Ethnic origin

Shared Care Network clearly advocates a same-race policy. The essence of good quality care is continuity. We believe that this can only be achieved if a same-race policy is in operation. Where schemes are unable to achieve this it is suggested that, as a minimum, link families should be given race equality training and fully briefed on the child's background and culture. The following is a summary of the same-race policy. See the **Policy statements section** at the end of the guide for the complete policy.

Same-race placements

Shared Care Network actively promotes same-race placements which provide continuity between the child's own home, and the short-term placement. This must always be our primary aim.

Where this is not possible, the child should be placed with another black community rather than a white family. Carers should be given race awareness training and full information on the child with whom they are matched, including information on their beliefs. They should also receive full back-up and support. Carers should respect the child's cultural and religious needs and offer care that reflects this.

Services should be continually encouraging the wider recruitment of carers from minority ethnic groups. Only by ensuring that there is a sufficient pool of carers from these groups can services work towards same-race placements for the majority of children and adults.

Life-style

Information about the carer's and child's life-style should be obtained:

- Does the carer smoke?
- Are there any pets in the home?
- Is this what the child is accustomed to?
- Is the carer a meat eater or vegetarian?
- Does the child prefer indoor/outdoor activities, to be active or calm, a structured or flexible daily routine?

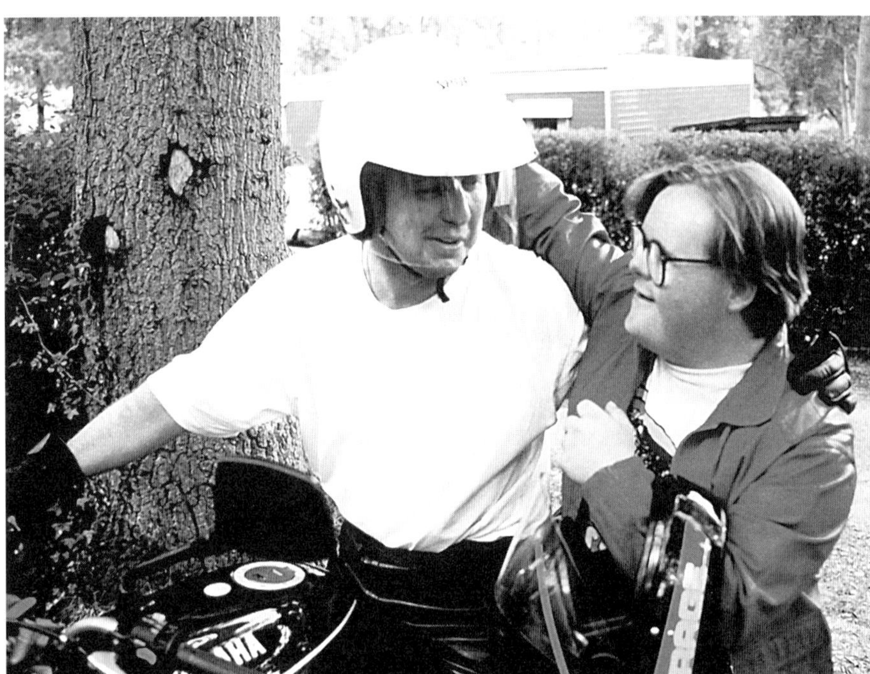

Religion

Carers should be willing to respect the child's religious beliefs and provide appropriate diets which reflect the child's religious or cultural background.

The carer's environment

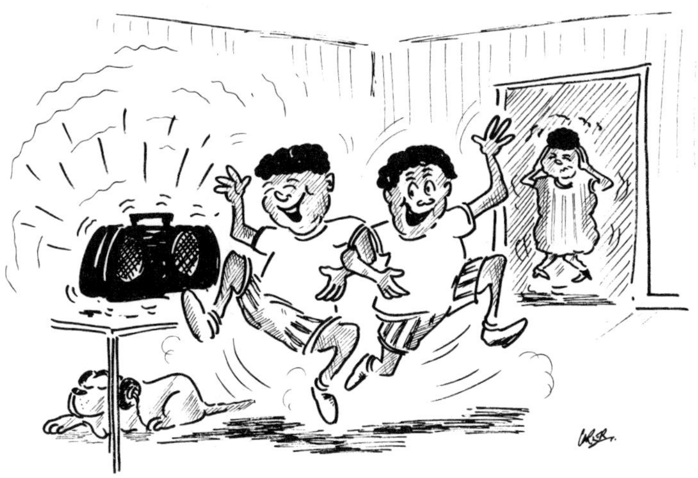

The carer's ability to look after and lift children with severe physical disabilities should be assessed in addition to practical issues. For example, is the carer's home accessible for wheelchairs? If carers are classed as employees there is a legal requirement to assess the carer's environment (see **Shared Care Network Lifting and Handling Policy** in the **Policy statements** section).

The carer's experience

Consideration should be given to the carer's ability to learn and continue training, especially if a child has complex medical needs or challenging behaviour.

Other factors which need to be considered when matching are:

- the amount of time the carers could offer and their flexibility;
- the geographic location – travel arrangements will need to be considered;
- the child's care needs which include physical, psychological and emotional needs;
- the ability of the carer to work in partnership with the particular family – both children and parents;

- the ability of the carer's immediate family to cope with the needs of the proposed child.

A quality service ensures consistency of care and reinforces the child's identity. This should be borne in mind throughout the matching process.

All of the needs of the individuals should be acknowledged. Essentially it is a process of partnership and should involve an honest exchange of information between everyone involved. Workers should maintain contact with those concerned and respond to expressed anxieties. It should be acknowledged that people have a right to withdraw or express concern during introductory periods without fear of jeopardising any future links. If a link ends at any time it is important to acknowledge the contribution of all parties and highlight the positive aspects.

See also Section 10, **Training and support for carers**, 'When placements end', page 126.

The number of links per carer

The 1989 Children Act states under Paragraph 2 and 3 of Schedule 7 that the usual fostering limit should be three children. The limit does not apply if the children are siblings.

It is clearly not good practice to overburden carers. We have yet to find examples of good practice that exceed five links per carer. This is based on carers who are available all year round; carers with less availability should have proportionately fewer links.

Agreements

At the end of the matching process and once introductory meetings have taken place it is important to draw up a placement agreement for the child. An example of an agreement drawn up by Warwickshire Family Link is shown below.

Written placement agreement form

1. As required by the 1989 Children Act, this is a written agreement between:

   (Parents' names)

   (Address) Date of birth

   Parents of (child's name) School

   and: (Carers' names)

   (Address) GP

   and/or (Agency name and address) Tel

   Setting up a short-term care agreement for one year from .... to ....

   Up to .... days/nights = in total .... hours

2. This agreement will be reviewed after three months, as required by the 1989 Children Act and then every six months, first review being in: and subsequent review in:

3. The expectations of (child's name) .... and his/her parents are that short stays/visits will be at approximately .... intervals.

4. Arrangements will be made as follows, for example, parents phoning to ask for particular dates/carers/project offering particular dates? Planning a series of dates in advance? A combination of these?

   Transport arrangements are agreed as follows:

   In an emergency (if parents or wider family cannot care for child) we agree that:

   Will the short stay always be offered in the carer's home, or sometimes in the child's own home?

5.(a) (child's name) ....'s parents understand that although (carers) will do their best to be available on the dates needed, this will not always be possible.

5.(b) In the event that (child's name) .... is ill, and the short stay cannot therefore go ahead, alternative arrangements will be made wherever possible.

6. (child's name) has now had .... introductory visits.

7. Carers/project staff have read (child's name) ....'s profile and understand that the following is very important in his/her care:

Parents and carers/key worker agree to discuss any issues or difficulties together. Either is welcome to discuss these with scheme/project leader at any time.

8. We believe that (child's name) .... agrees to follow this arrangement because:

9. Parents have signed the medical consent form and agree to send medication for each stay with prescription labels giving name, dosage and times.

10. Scheme only – parents have signed Parents' Undertakings. Carers have signed the Carers' Undertaking (copies to parents, social worker, scheme coordinator).

11. Signed

Parents

Carers/key worker

Child

Child's social worker tel

Scheme coordinator tel

Parents, carers/key worker, social worker and scheme coordinator/ project leader all have a copy of this agreement (child's social worker completes a variation form on this date also authorising a series of short stays for a year).

Matching detail form

1. Name of child
2. Sex
3. Address of child
4. Child's date of birth
5. Age
6. (a) Has child's family any preference regarding race/religion/culture of support family? Yes/No

   (b) If yes: (i) Please specify preference

   (ii) Would other race/religion/culture be acceptable? Yes/No

   (iii) If yes, what?
7. (a) What is your child's primary need?

   (b) Does he/she have any other special needs (for example, sight/hearing difficulties)? Yes/No

   If yes, what are these?
8. Does your child have any medical needs (for example, epilepsy, tube feeding, suction)? Yes/No

   If yes, please refer to detailed forms in *Towards a healthy future.*
9. (a) Can your child walk independently? Yes/No

   (b) If not, please tell us what your child is able to do.
10. (a) Can you tell us a little about your child's behaviour?

Is he/she:	Quiet?	Yes/No
	Aggressive?	Yes/No
	Easy going?	Yes/No
	Demanding of your time/attention?	Yes/No

(b) Please tell us anything else about your child's behaviour which will help us find the right support family.

(c) What reactions do you experience in caring for your child?

Tiredness	Yes/No
Joy	Yes/No
Frustration	Yes/No
Satisfaction	Yes/No
Fulfilment	Yes/No
Anger	Yes/No

(d) Please tell us anything else about what you feel in caring for your child.

11. (a) Finally, please tell us about the things your child can do. For example, can he/she:

Feed him/herself?	Yes/No
Go to the toilet?	Yes/No
Make known his/her wants or needs?	Yes/No

(b) Please add anything else about what your child can do.

Now that we have an idea of your child's needs, we can move on to what the scheme could do for both him/her and you!

12. (a) Is your child currently receiving any short-term care or day care? Yes/No

(b) If yes, what, where and how often?

13. Can you think of any problems which have arisen before which you think we should look out for (such as settling down difficulties, homesickness, difficult behaviour when he/she comes home)?

14. Have you got any ideas yet on how you would like to use the scheme? (For example, how many days per week? how long each time? It doesn't matter if you are not yet absolutely clear.)

15. (a) Has your child any particular cultural, religious or dietary needs which you would like us to try and match? Yes/No

    (b) If yes, what are these?

16. Are there any other things you think we need to remember when looking for a support family for you and your child?

17. Finally, so that the support family understand how best to look after your child, they need the information on this form. Is that OK?
    Yes/No

18. Once we have a support family which may be able to help, where would you like to meet them?

Anywhere (no preference)	Yes/No
At the project	Yes/No
At your home	Yes/No
At their home	Yes/No
Somewhere else	Yes/No

19. We will be trying to find a family who live locally. If this is not possible, is transport likely to be a difficulty for you? Yes/No

20. Please detail any special equipment which will need to go with your child, for example, feeding or bathing aids.

21. Is there anything else you'd like to tell us at this stage?

Reviewing and monitoring placements

8

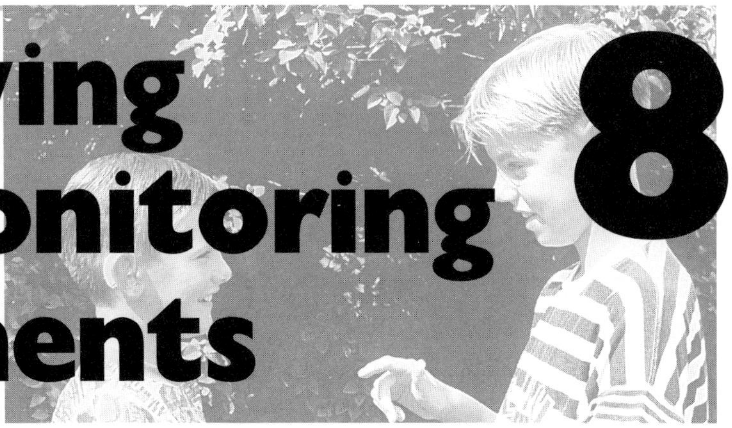

In this section issues around reviewing and monitoring placements are considered and the new regulations regarding reviews and visits outlined. The following issues will also be explored:

- the welfare of children using multiple services;
- who should call review meetings;
- the purpose of reviewing children and families;
- preparing children for review meetings;
- preparing parents and carers for review meetings;
- the content of reviews;
- who should attend review meetings;
- where and when should reviews take place;
- complaints;
- transition plans.

Legislation and guidance

5. For regulation 11 of the Review of Children's Cases Regulations 1991(d) (application of Regulations to short periods) there shall be substituted the following regulation:

11.(1) This regulation applies to cases in which a responsible authority has arranged that a child should be looked after or provided with accommodation for a series of short periods at the same place and the arrangement is such that no single period is to last for more than four weeks and the total duration of the periods is not to exceed 120 days in any period of 12 months.

(2) Regulation 3 shall not apply to a case to which this regulation applies, but instead:

(a) each such case is first to be reviewed within 3 months of the beginning of the first of the short periods;

(b) if the case continues, the second review shall be carried out not more than 6 months after the first; and

(c) thereafter, if the case continues, subsequent reviews shall be carried out not more than 6 months after the date of the previous review.

(3) For the purposes of Regulation 6, a child shall be treated as continuing to be looked after or provided with accommodation throughout the period that this regulation applies to his case. (1995 Children [Short-term Placements] [Miscellaneous Amendments] Regulations)

Introduction

In August 1995 relaxation of the requirements governing short-term care placements were introduced. Shared Care Network had actively lobbied the Department of Health and welcomed most of the amendments. The new regulations relating to short-term care are outlined above. The implications of these in relation to visits and reviews are discussed below.

Visits and reviews of placements

The 1989 Children Act only concerns regulations for placements over 24 hours long. It is, however, not good practice to treat stays of under 24 hours as being outside the regulations as this would create a two-tier system with the danger that some users will resist crossing the 24 hour barrier in order to avoid being subject to the full review procedure. To do so would also mean that some children who have large amounts of care will remain outside the review system, because no period of care is 24 hours or longer.

Under the new regulations, the Act requires that a child is visited within the first seven placement days (that is, seven days when the child is actually in placement) or before the first review, whichever is the sooner. Visiting is one way of safeguarding the welfare of children who are placed away from home and should not just be seen as a statutory requirement. Visits should be carried out by the social worker. Placements should be reviewed within three months of the commencement of the placement, then at six-monthly intervals thereafter.

The new regulations move the limit for short-term care to 120 days in a 12-month period instead of 90 days, although it is unlikely that many schemes will be able to fund 120 days care a year. The 90-day limit is still applicable in Northern Ireland. Shared Care Network has, however, actively lobbied against raising the limit to 120 days. Social workers are advised to be extremely cautious should a child's use of the service approach this limit.

It may on occasion be necessary to call a planning meeting outside the review process. The 'Looking after children' procedure may be useful in relation to this in particular cases.

What about children using multiple services?

Where children are using more than one service which offers short-term care, well-planned regular reviews of placement are essential so that services are coordinated and good childcare practice is ensured.

Representatives from each of the services involved should be invited to a single review where the use of all relevant services is discussed. The Audit Commission's report, *Seen but not heard* (1994), clearly states that there is a greater need for coordinated reviews between agencies. In addition Standard 3 outlined in the Social Services Inspectorate report, *Removing barriers for disabled children* (SSI, 1998a) states: "disabled children and their families receive services that are timely, responsive to their needs and which have been identified through an effective, co-ordinated multi-disciplinary process".

Who should call the review meetings?

It is good practice for scheme coordinators to call review meetings, bearing in mind that they arranged the placements. However, if a child is accommodated the local authority's social worker for the child should undertake this task unless agreement has been designated to the scheme coordinator. It is recognised that not all children will have a social worker and in these cases there is little choice but for the scheme coordinator to call the meeting. An efficient system for scheduling meetings should be in place to prevent reviews of placement being overlooked.

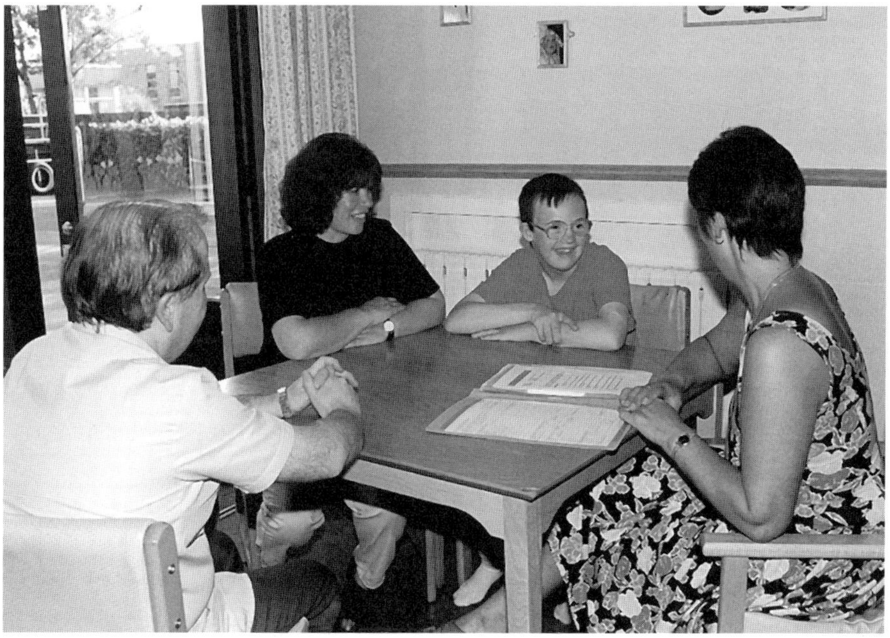

Why review children and families?

- To ensure the placement is promoting the welfare of the child.
- To explore the child's views about the placement.
- To meet the regulations.
- To examine the needs of the child, family, siblings and carers and assess how far these are being met.
- To review current written agreements and update them and to revise the childcare plan.
- If no other reviews are taking place, to look at unmet need and either address the issues or refer to other agencies. This could be done at a planning meeting.

Reviews of placement should not be seen as only dealing with problems. Professionals should use them as a chance to give positive feedback to all parties. It should be possible for any interested party to call a review at any time.

Preparing children for review meetings

For children to be involved in their reviews of placement in a meaningful way it is important to give them an opportunity to communicate their views in a neutral setting to someone who does not have a vested interest in the placement continuing (see Section 6 on **Consulting children, parents and carers**).

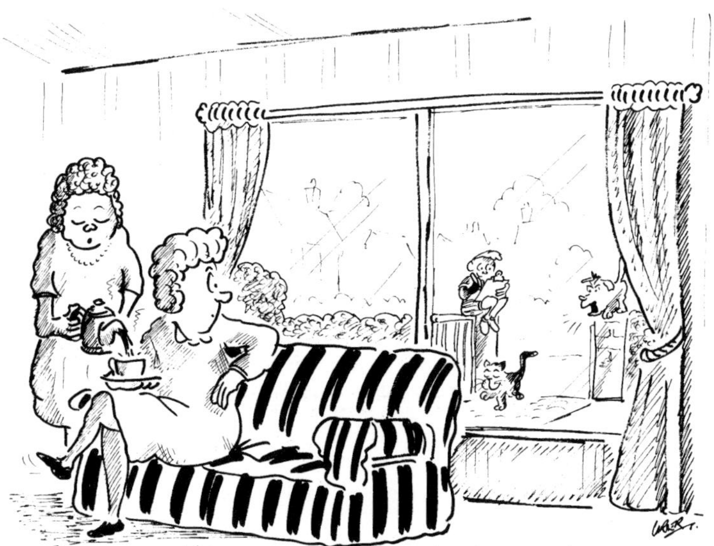

He's reviewing and Monitoring us Himself

This could be done in school, or through appropriate leisure services, for example, after school clubs, by youth workers, teachers, welfare assistants, escorts – providing they have a good relationship with the child. For this to work effectively, the person will need to be fully briefed on the process, including issues of confidentiality. The child needs to be clear about what his/her role will be in the review meeting and it is important that the person chairing the meeting takes account of the child's views. The child should also be made aware of any decisions that are made and it should be ensured that s/he is happy with these.

Preparing parents and carers for review meetings

Experience shows that people can find reviews of placement intimidating. It is important, therefore, that parents and carers are prepared for what is essentially a formal meeting. Including parents in the planning may be beneficial, giving them choice of time, venue and who, as far as possible, should be invited. This may be done through:

- pre-review visits to discuss the issues that may arise;
- written information asking for comments;
- questionnaires.

Well-handled reviews will allow less assertive users or link carers to raise issues of concern. The importance of maintaining confidentiality should be emphasised to all parties.

What should the review cover?

The following issues should be discussed.

- To what extent does the childcare plan continue to be relevant?
- Is the placement appropriate?
- Are the practical arrangements for the placement (for example, transport and equipment) working?
- Is the level and frequency of breaks adequate, too much or too little?
- What are the clear benefits to the child and what is this based on?
- What benefits does this offer to the family and is it the most appropriate service to use?
- Are there any disadvantages to the family including siblings?
- What are the benefits/disadvantages to carers?

Families should always get copies of review decisions in a language appropriate to them. Reviews of placement should be conducted in a way that takes account of race, gender, culture and so on.

Who should be invited to the review?

Below are listed the people who should attend review meetings.

- the child or young person, following appropriate preparation;
- the parents and the link family;
- friend or advocate, if available;
- the child's social worker;
- the link worker;
- someone independent of the placement to chair the meeting, for example, a reviewing officer;
- in addition, it may be appropriate to involve siblings, key professionals and any one else significantly involved in the child's life;
- an interpreter.

Voluntary agencies cannot call statutory reviews. A representative of the local authority must be present and agree to any action plan.

Where and when should reviews of placement take place?

The same types of considerations apply to setting review meetings as they do for other training or assessment events. That is:

- a comfortable, accessible venue, ideally chosen by the family;

- meetings should be at a time when all concerned can attend, for example, after school or at a time when parents are not at work.

Complaints

Should parents express dissatisfaction with the way plans for the child's care are being implemented, workers should make efforts to deal with the complaint in an informal manner. Parents should already have received information about the agency's complaints procedures and been given the appropriate information and forms and these should be drawn to their attention if they are still dissatisfied with the service (for an example, see page 117 on reviewing the approval of carers).

Transition plans

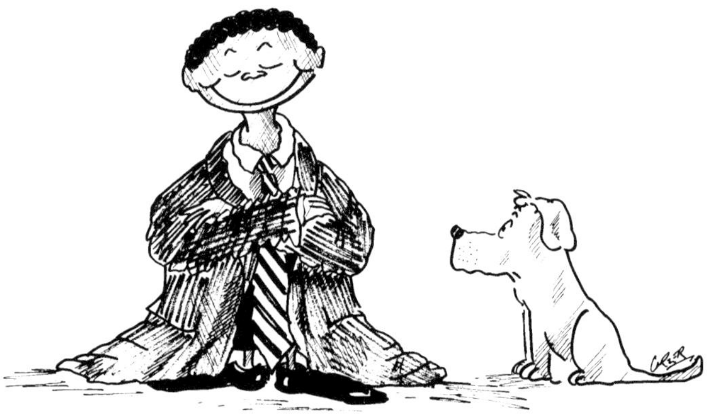

The transition to adulthood can be confusing, or at worst, traumatic, for both young people and carers. There can be several agencies involved, as well as specialists within these agencies, who may understand little about each other's services. Failure to plan thoroughly and examine the options available can lead to carers receiving little or no support or losing out financially. Equally, young people may be placed in settings that do not best meet their needs.

Legal responsibilities

The principal aim of Sections 5 and 6 of the 1986 Disabled Persons Act is the facilitation of the smooth transition of young people with disabilities from full-time education to adulthood. The key task in achieving this is the identification of the young person's needs before they leave full-time education.

Young people with special needs should receive a formal statement of their needs by the local education authority when they reach 14 years of age and again before they reach 16. This enables their needs to be assessed and plans made to meet these needs. The local education authority is required to notify the social services department of any disabled young person who will be leaving school in the next eight to 12 months.

The 1993 Education Act provides for this very careful reviewing procedure and carers should ensure that, where appropriate, there is cooperation between the local education authority and the relevant social services department. This is obviously of vital importance if the young person is assessed as having a disability along with possible care needs into adulthood.

When public funding is required for adults, the local authority will have sole responsibility for providing care and accommodation in the community. This applies to those persons whom it assesses as being in need of care and attention by reason of age, illness, disability and so on. These obligations were laid down by Part III of the 1948 National Assistance Act (as amended by the 1992 Community Care [Residential Accommodation] Act).

Social services departments are guided by the 1990 National Health Service and Community Care Act and the 1968 Social Worker (Scotland) Act, to identify 18 years old as the age when a young person changes from being a child to being an adult. Social services departments should start planning for this transfer at least a year before it is due to happen.

The children and young people's services of a local authority could, in certain circumstances, continue to offer services to an individual up to the age of 21. This could apply if the individual was 'looked after' after the age of 15.

It is vital to ensure that the local authority is aware of and meeting its assessment and planning responsibilities before any discussion can begin about whether the child will continue to need a family placement.

The young person

- A 'community care' assessment of the young person's needs should be undertaken by the social services department.
- A series of questions need to be asked including:
  - Will the young person continue to require family or residential short-term care?
  - Is an adult placement in the best interests of the young person?
  - If so, are the current carers considered to be the best people to meet these needs?
  - Does the young person want to continue to receive care from his/her carer/s?
  - Have all the possible options and alternatives been considered?

The support carer/s

A similar set of questions need to be considered.

- Do the carers want to continue to offer care to the young person?
- Has the adult placement service assessed them as suitable carers for a young adult?
- Are they aware of the possible implications of adulthood – particularly in terms of medical treatment, personal care and risk assessment?
- Are they aware of all the possible placement options for the young person?
- Are they willing to make a long-term commitment?
- Do the carers want to become part of an adult placement scheme?
- They are under no obligation to join a scheme but are they aware of the pitfalls involved in standing alone, for example, being seen as an independent provider, the need for a contract with the local authority and different payment systems?
- Are they clear about the tax and benefit implications of the different options?
- Adult placement schemes can offer financial support, but will it be adequate for them?
- Are the carers wishing to provide care for more than 28 days a year? If so they need to register under the 1991 Registered Homes (Amendment) Act.
- Are they offering 'board and personal care'? If they have cared for the young person for less than five years they will need to register under the 1991 Registered Homes (Amendment) Act.

- Are they aware of the implications of the Registered Homes (Amendment) Act? (The requirements can be quite institutional but registration enables them to offer care for up to three people throughout the year.)

A competent adult placement worker will guide the carers through registration under the Registered Homes (Amendment) Act and hopefully the homely, domestic nature that is the very essence of family placement can continue.

If it is decided that it is not in the young person's best interests to continue with the original carer:

- Approach the adult care scheme to see what alternative carers are available. (This would normally be under the local authority that initially authorised and funded the shared care.)
- Work alongside the adult scheme and the individual's care manager in order to ensure the best placement is found.

Good adult placement schemes will offer support, financial advice, knowledge of local adult services, training and access to other adult carers. Most authorities have such schemes while those that do not, or have a shortage of carers, can approach neighbouring schemes to see if they are able to provide a service.

The National Association of Adult Placement Services (NAAPS) publishes a directory of adult placement schemes in the UK. Shared Care Network's own directory also includes some short-term adult services.

Reviewing the approval of carers

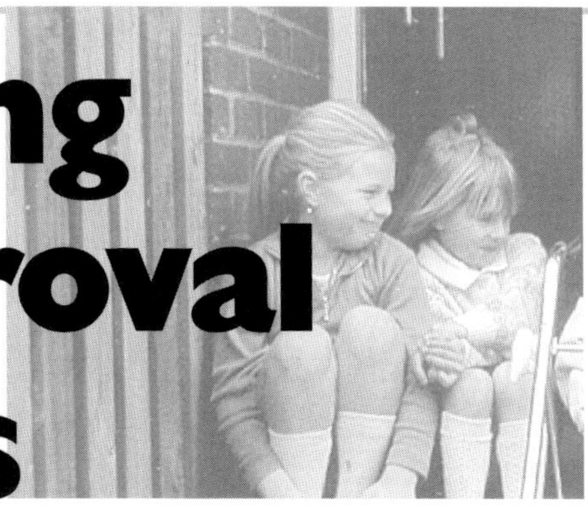

9

The aim of this section is to consider some of the issues around reviewing the approval of carers. The following areas will be discussed:

- the purpose of reviewing carers;
- the content of reviews;
- notification;
- challenging decisions.

Legislation and guidance

Authorities are required by Regulation 4 to review the approval of foster parents at least once a year. Reviews should focus on the foster parent rather than the current placement and should, if possible, be carried out by a social worker with responsibility to the fostering service that may not be the social worker of a child in placement. Consultation would then of course be necessary to establish how the placement is working and what the child and his parents' views on this are. A review should include a visit to the foster home, discussion with the foster parent and the child, and generally meeting other members of the household. It should be an opportunity for airing and discussion of the foster parent's view of the service offered by the authority and of the foster parent's own experience and any difficulties arising. (1989 Children Act Guidance and Regulations, Vol 3, Sections 3.44-3.45)

Introduction

The legal requirements outlined above highlight the status of short-term carers as foster carers. As such, local authorities and voluntary agencies have clear responsibilities towards them. In this section the steps involved in reviewing the approval of carers are outlined and consideration given as to how carers may challenge a review decision with which they are unhappy.

Why review carers?

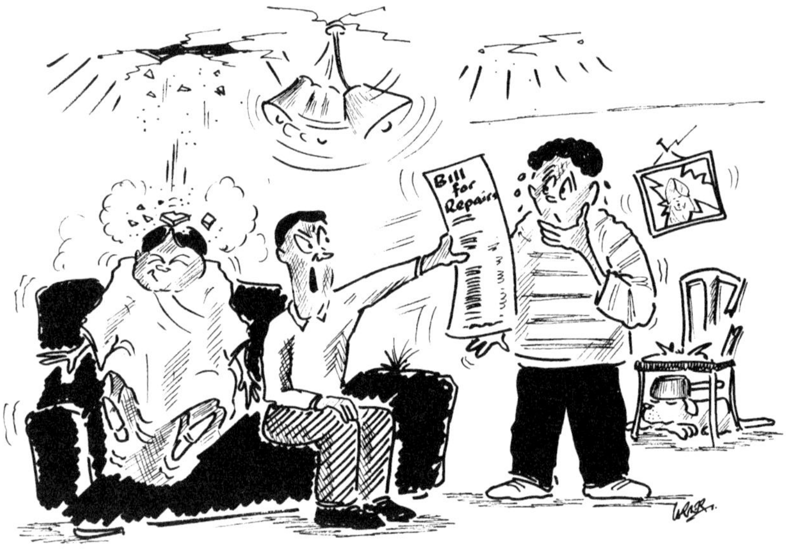

Carers' reviews are about maintaining and developing carers' skills and giving them an opportunity to voice their concerns.

The content of reviews

Good reapproval meetings should address quality issues and look at carers' training needs and the best ways to meet them.

Discussion should cover the following issues:

- major changes in carers' circumstances;
- equipment/access needs;
- the carer's children;
- what they enjoy about caring;
- what has been the most difficult experience;
- how they have found working with families;
- what sort of children they think they are best linked with;
- if they are happy providing the level of service they currently offer;
- what use they make currently in terms of training/ carers' groups;
- what other training or support would be useful;
- practical issues – update police checks/medicals;
- personal aspirations.

The same considerations should be given to the venue, timing, and so on, of visits as outlined in the section on reviewing placements above.

Consulting families

Under the Act, social workers are required to consult with all families of children currently linked to the carer and to any children's families who were linked within the previous 12 months. The purpose of this is to give them an opportunity to comment on the care they have received and to raise any issues of concern. It is important in this letter to reassure families that this is a statutory requirement.

Since the introduction of the Act, reviews have been seen as burdensome, time-consuming and excessively bureaucratic. However, they are essential to providing a good quality service, and should be accessible and understandable to all concerned.

Notification of the review

Carers should receive a copy of their report in writing before formal reapproval takes place, and be given a chance to comment. Once the carer is reapproved they should receive a formal letter outlining the terms of reapproval.

Challenging decisions

These requirements to review are fairly recent and for some carers the possibility, although unlikely, of having their registration terminated can cause anxiety. They should, therefore, have maximum advice, if this is even a remote possibility, along with the areas of concern in writing.

In Volume 3 of the 1989 Children Act Guidance and Regulations, it is suggested that under the 1989 Children Act there is no statutory provision for carers to have access to a procedure to make representations or a complaint on their own behalf except in connection with decisions about the usual fostering limit. It states, however, that carers should be able to make representations about disputes and discuss facts connected with other aspects of their service as carers. These may include disputes about the care of a child, dissatisfaction with the support or services provided by the authority and requests for review of decisions such as refusal of approval, termination of approval or termination of a placement. Responsible authorities may therefore wish to extend their statutory 1989 Children Act complaints procedures to include complaints made by carers on their own behalf.

! *Note: Although there are differences in the way carers and agency employees are treated in regard to grievances and complaints procedures, carers should be fully aware of the local arrangement pertaining to them.*

The following is an example of a method used by a service in Dudley to invite comment.

Your comments are welcome!

Are you unhappy about any decision we have made?

Do you want to tell us about something that we should be proud of?

Do you just want to tell us about something?

Then use our comments form! The children with our service want to hear from you whether you have something good or bad to say about us.

This is not the official complaints or grievance procedure but it does give us the chance to look informally at issues without fear of anything happening to the individuals involved. We would hope that it gives us better feedback from you, and that we can improve the way we do things.

There should be a form to use with this leaflet. If not please ring us
on .... and we will forward it to you.

Training and support for carers 10

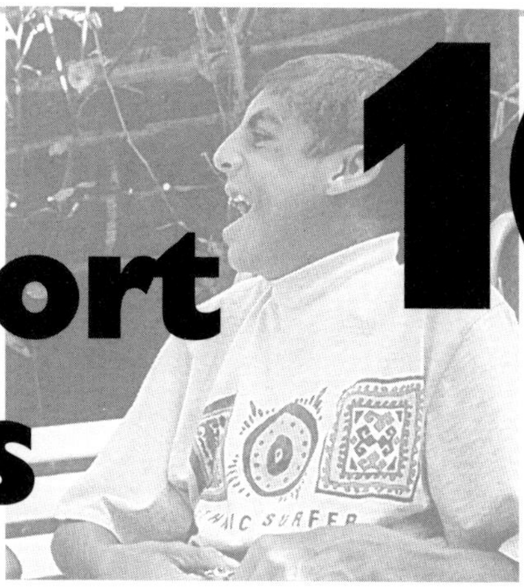

This section addresses the training and support needs of carers with particular reference to the following:

- assessing carers' training needs;
- who should provide the training;
- what training should be offered;
- support for carers via support groups, support from professionals and newsletters;
- when placements end;
- saying thank you and recognising contributions of carers.

Legislation and guidance

Social workers need access to appropriate training resources to meet the needs of foster parents.... The help of health professionals should be sought in local training schemes.... Reading matter should also be available to foster parents. All training should aim to enable foster parents to help and work with children in the context of a multi-racial society and to develop positive attitudes towards less advantaged groups. Foster parents need support and help with difficulties that arise from the special demands of the fostering role, in addition to help that may be needed in connection with the care of a particular child.... Authorities should ensure that appropriate support, advice and assistance are provided to the foster parent and foster family. (1989 Children Act Guidance and Regulations, Vol 3, Section 3.55)

Introduction

In an earlier section, preparation of carers was considered. Preparation gives carers a basic grounding in disability/ childcare issues in readiness for a child's stay. Training, however, is intended to develop carers' skills and knowledge further and should be ongoing. This section begins with ways to find out what carers need to know and considers ways of making carers feel valued.

Assessing carers' training needs

The training and development needs of carers should be addressed throughout their careers as carers.

Carers who come forward to offer short-term care will have had very different experiences. Annual reviews provide an ideal opportunity to assess carers' strengths and to determine in which areas they feel less well equipped. They offer the chance to look at carers' training needs and ways in which these can be met.

While it is recommended that preparation sessions are made mandatory, ongoing training should be seen as a development programme which is offered to carers and is optional. Services could choose to require carers to attend a certain number of ongoing training sessions but this would need to be outlined in the foster placement agreement. For example, to safeguard carers, you may expect their attendance at a workshop about how to deal with allegations of abuse. Below is an example of a letter which urges carers to attend a meeting on HIV/AIDS.

Dear Carer

Re: HIV/AIDS AWARENESS TRAINING

Two training sessions have been arranged on HIV/AIDS awareness. You are strongly urged to attend one of these meetings or to indicate that you have attended similar training elsewhere, for example, via your employment. It is considered to be essential that all the scheme's carers have received relevant information and training regarding this very sensitive health matter and that safe practices are adopted which also offer protection against Hepatitis. The training is offered by a professional trainer who is employed by the Health Promotion Service.

The meetings will be held at the .... A map is enclosed. The first session will be on Wednesday 15 June at 7.30pm. The second session will be on Thursday 23 June at 10am-12noon. Please complete the slip attached and return it to the office as soon as possible using the enclosed stamped addressed envelope. Those carers unable to attend these sessions will be invited to attend one later in the year.

Yours sincerely

Please tick the appropriate box. I/we will be able to attend the session:

June 15 evening ❐

June 23 morning ❐

I have received training awareness elsewhere ❐

Signed .... Date ....

The training offered by schemes gives many carers the grounding and confidence to go on to pursue professional careers in the field of social care and should never be undervalued.

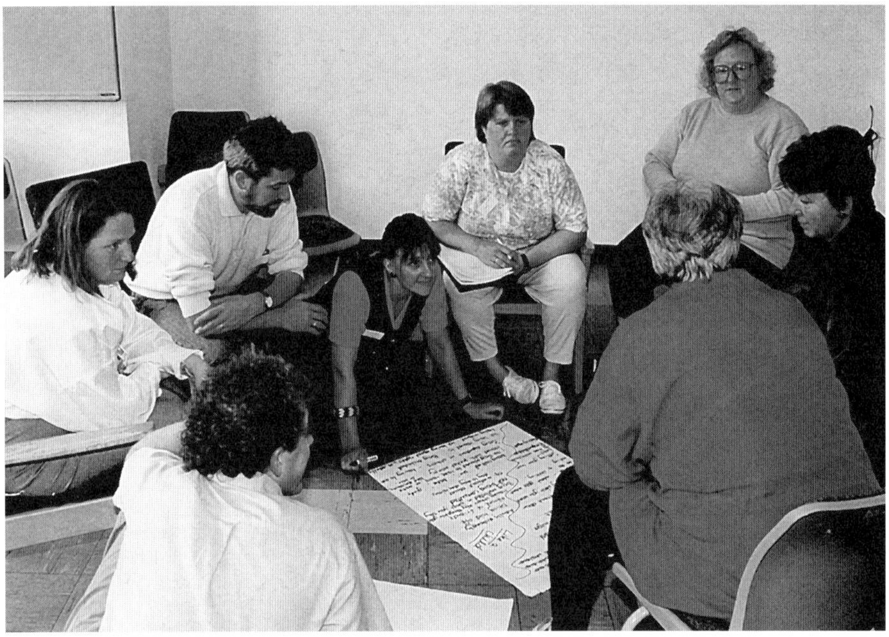

Who should provide the training?

Scheme organisers are responsible for ensuring that training is made available; they are not responsible for carrying out all of the training. If possible, plug into existing training, look at what exists locally and tap into it. For example, use courses offered to foster carers or ones available at local colleges or other agencies such as the Workers Educational Association or social services training departments. The development of NVQ courses for foster carers is welcome and it is important that short-term carers have access to the same opportunities.

What training should be offered?

An outline of the training topics which would be important for short-term carers is presented below.

- Understanding of disability/civil rights including the 1995 Disability Discrimination Act
- First Aid/Epilepsy
- Risk assessments
- HIV and AIDS
- Confidentiality
- Emerging sexuality
- Makaton/Total Communication
- Safety in the home
- Race awareness
- Managing challenging behaviour
- Safe caring – protecting carers and children
- Toys and play
- Working with severe sensory impairment
- Autism
- Age appropriateness
- Disability awareness
- Moving and handling
- Providing intimate care
- Complex healthcare
- Services and support for disabled children (an overview of current arrangements under the 1989 Children Act, the 1993 Education Act and the 1986 Disabled Persons Act)
- Assertiveness training (very useful for carers who find it hard to say no to families even when it is inconvenient)

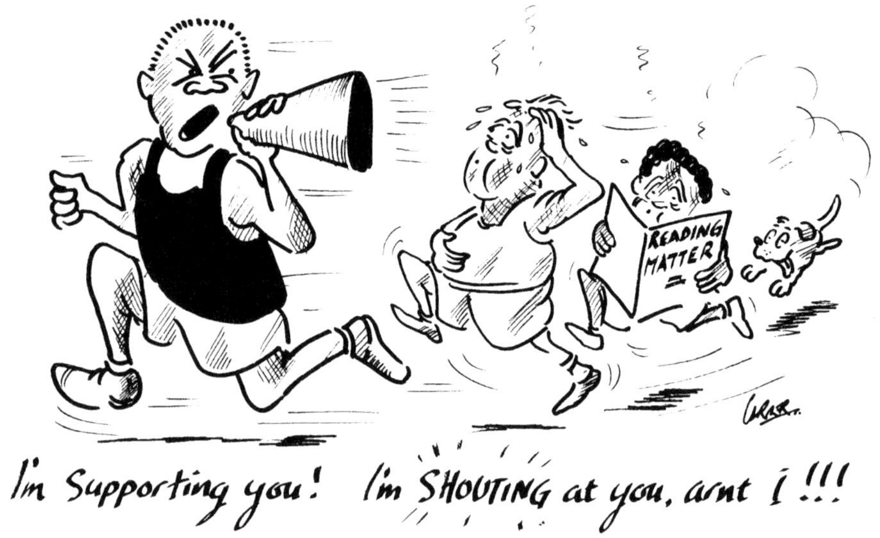

Support for carers

Support for carers is extremely important and can be offered through a variety of sources.

Carers' support groups

During the preparation stages many carers will have formed natural groups which often become their own informal support group. If this does not occur the agency may need to step in to take the initiative. Throughout the life of a group there may be low points and scheme workers may need to step in to revive it. Support groups can take the form of meetings or less formally via social events held for carers. One option may be to link carers into parents' support groups if they exist locally. You may also consider setting up specific groups, for example, a black carers' and/or Asian carers' group.

Support from professionals

Regular contact with the link worker allows the carer to air any concerns or difficulties they may be experiencing. Home visits may not always be possible but a telephone call to see how things are going can offer carers a feeling of support. The minimum level of contact that will be offered should be written into the foster care agreement. A telephone survey of support carers carried out by Shared Care Network (Newitt et al, 1997) indicated that, on the whole, carers felt well supported by their scheme. Overall, 95% of carers were happy with the support they received from the service. However, one quarter of respondents did not know about an emergency back-up system where it existed. Where problems did arise, most (62%) said they would turn to the scheme worker.

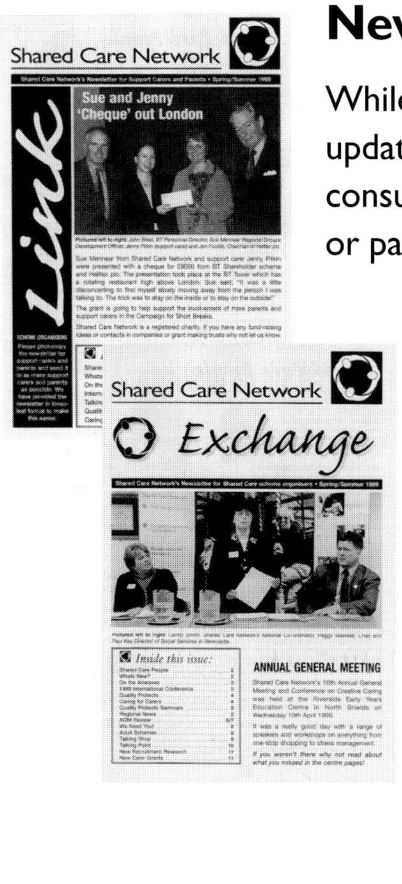

Newsletters

While newsletters are a good way to keep people updated about the scheme they can be very time consuming to put together. If possible, encourage carers or parents to take on this task.

Support when things go wrong

It is important that all services have comprehensive child protection procedures in place. Carers should be clear about how these operate and be told what they can expect from the agency if allegations are made against them. It is particularly important that carers should know that if their care practices are subject to enquiry, they will be given support by one worker and the child's interest will be presented by another worker.

When placements end

It should be recognised that links are a phase in someone's life and will naturally come to an end at some point. Support and reassurance should be given to the people involved to help them through the change.

Relationships end for a variety of reasons and the task is to understand the reasons and assist those involved to work through the process.

A placement may end amid allegations of abuse or irregularities and agencies must have written procedures for the carer, user and family.

Where bereavement occurs, carers should be offered counselling or be put in touch with relevant organisations such as Cruse (Bereavement Care).

Where placements end on a difficult note it would be useful to bring all the parties together for two reasons:

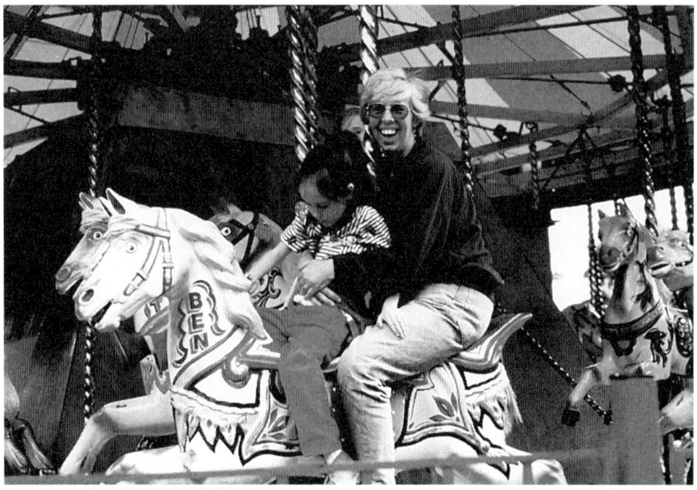

- to arrange a positive ending for the child, for example, a favourite outing;
- to learn the lessons of the placement so that the family and carer can move positively to the next placement.

It is important to record the positive aspects of the placement and the extent to which progress has been made. The carer may be able to provide useful information to consider when organising the next placement for the child.

Any end of placement discussions should cover the following:

- what the carer found rewarding;
- what the carer found difficult;
- what was the impact of the placement on the carer's children;
- whether the placement matched the carer's strengths and abilities;
- what the agency should have provided and could provide in the future.

Saying thank you

Most carers offer their services, not for financial reasons, but because they feel they are making an important contribution. It is important for the agency to recognise this formally from time to time and also to pass on positive comments received from users or parents.

Quality assurance in family-based shared care schemes

11

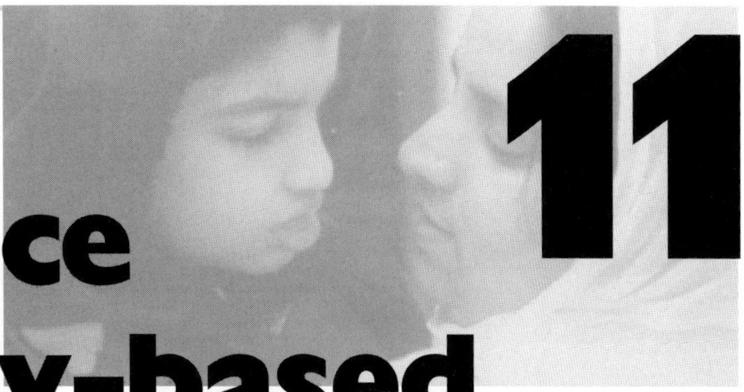

This section will look at how to:

- provide some specific input on current quality issues and on the importance of quality;
- use some broad indicators to begin to measure quality;
- look at setting up specific quality measures and standards in relation to shared care schemes;
- provide one way of looking at quality in a specific service which can be adopted.

Legislation and guidance

Work with children with disabilities in the 1989 Children Act should be based on the following principles:

- *the welfare of the child should be safeguarded and promoted by those providing services;*
- *a primary aim should be to promote access for all children to the same range of services;*
- *children with disabilities are children first;*
- *recognition of the importance of parents and families in children's lives;*
- *partnership between parents and local authorities and other agencies; and*
- *the views of children and parents should be sought and taken into account. (1989 Children Act, Vol 6, Section 1.6)*

Introduction

There are many services offering short-term care to children and the number of people using family-based care is increasing, but how can services be sure that they are providing what is best for children and families? This section begins by identifying some basic indicators of quality and goes on to how these can be interpreted.

Indicators of quality

Jones (1989) identified some factors which can be used to indicate the quality of the service provided which should be considered when carrying out an evaluation study.

1 Flexibility and availability of the service

For example, how long it takes to provide a regular link for a child, how quickly the service can respond in a crisis and how responsive the service can be to children and situations that do not fit any of the usual categories.

2 Representation and penetration

For example, how does the demographic mix of the children provided with short-term care match the demographic mix of the area as a whole? Is the service reaching out to families who need the service the most?

3 Quality of linking

For example, are children's families being provided with the sort of carer family they asked for and are carer families being asked to take on the sort of children they agreed to take when they were approved? Are children's needs being matched with carer families' skills? Is culture considered during the matching processes?

4 Quality of care given in a link

For example, is the quality of care in accordance with accepted standards of 'good enough parenting' and is the quality of the care in accordance with the accepted codes of practice within short-term care generally?

Unfortunately, to be able to evaluate the quality of care being provided, terms like *good enough parenting* need to be defined. Below are some of the basic needs of children which should be met:

- **basic physical care** which includes warmth, shelter, adequate food and rest, grooming, hygiene and protection from danger;
- **affection** which includes physical contact, holding, stroking, cuddling and kissing, comforting, admiration, delight, tenderness, patience, time, making allowances for annoying behaviour, good companionship and approval;
- **security** which involves continuity of care, the expectation of continuing in the stable family unit, predictable environment, consistent patterns of care and daily routine, simple rules and consistent controls and harmonious family group;
- **stimulating innate potential** by praise, by encouraging curiosity and exploratory behaviour, by developing skills through responsiveness to questions and to play by promoting educational opportunities;
- **guidance and control** to teach adequate social behaviour which includes discipline within the child's understanding and capacity, and which requires patience and a model for the child to copy, for example, in honesty and concern and kindness for others (Cooper, 1985).

Setting up a quality framework

A quality framework begins by asking simple questions of any service. What are you trying to do? For whom? To what standard? It is important for all services to ask these questions and is an essential part of setting up a new service or reviewing one.

The language of quality is borrowed from the world of commerce and can be seen as daunting – it needn't be, and what follows is a simple glossary.

Aims

A broad statement about what you are trying to do – no more than 20 words and agreed by everyone. For example,

> *To offer a family-based short-term care service to children and/or young people with disabilities who live in....*

Objectives

Objectives vary depending on the question, so:

a) What are you trying to achieve or are you currently achieving? (IMPACT OBJECTIVES or OUTCOMES) For example,

   To enable carers to offer children good experiences of short-term care.

b) What services do you provide to achieve the OUTCOMES or SERVICE OBJECTIVES. For example,

   To recruit local carers who will provide an appropriate service to families using the scheme.

c) What do we need to have in place to provide the service? (These are INPUT or LOGISTIC OBJECTIVES.) For example,

   To sustain approved carers by offering support through individual and/or group meetings. This will include clarifying the training needs at the carer's annual review.

Aims and objectives are important for assessing the quality of service offered and should be:

- set by the service staff in conjunction with stakeholders (that is, all who have an interest);
- written as statements of intent;
- clarified in terms of the numbers of people and time-scales;
- based on clear standards (usually defined by the Act);
- beneficial to both staff and managers;
- reassessed in the light of time and significant changes.

Good objectives are backed by good standards.

Setting standards

Standards should be SMART!

Specific

Measurable

Attainable

Realistic

Timed

and:

- agreed and understood by all staff;
- objective and unambiguous;
- a commitment which service users can always expect.

The difference between objectives and standards needs to be clearly understood. Objectives by their very nature can be woolly – so an objective for carers might be "to assess and review carers in line with the 1989 Children Act – and to present the assessment to the Panel for approval".

Standards in relation to assessment and review would be:

- assessments will be completed in a four-month period;
- carers will see a copy of their draft assessment and be able to comment on it;
- group preparation will be offered up to three times a year in [name of appropriate languages];
- carers will be required to attend up to three training sessions a year – one of which will focus on child protection.

It is important to remember that standards should be:

- achievable;
- flexible;
- measurable against the 1989 Children Act (if you need to set standards below the minimum set out in the Act, this needs to be a management decision with clear written reasons as to why this is the case).

Measuring standards

In 1996/97 Shared Care Network carried out a project looking at quality assurance in family-based short-term care. The aim was to promote models of quality assurance that involved the users of the service. Two models were used. The first involved using telephone questionnaires to obtain feedback from parents and support carers about the service. These questionnaires were piloted with 12 schemes and are available from Shared Care Network. *A question of quality* (Newitt, 1997) includes copies of the questionnaires and guidelines for their use. Many services have since used these tools to identify strengths and weaknesses in their services.

The second model used in the study is based on 'Quality action groups' which include service providers, support carers, users of services and their primary carers. Members of the group work together to look at the way the service is working and how it could be improved. For a review of both methods see *Quality counts* (Newitt et al, 1997).

This section has given an overview of quality assurance in family-based short-term care services. Indicators of quality have been outlined and suggestions made for setting up a quality framework and setting and measuring standards. By following these guidelines, schemes will be able to more accurately assess the quality of service they offer.

The example opposite illustrates how to identify practice areas and suggests standards and ways of checking they are met.

Carer recruitment and support

Item	Standard	Information source
Carer recruitment	There is clear evidence (such as a written plan) of planned approach to recruiting suitable carers.	Carer recruitment plan
	A variety of means (more than two) are used for publicising the service and the need for carers.	Carer recruitment records
	Analysis is done of the relative success of different methods of publicity and carer recruitment.	Carer recruitment policy/procedure
Carers receive training	All carers attend relevant training courses.	10 randomly selected carers' files
	All carers without such training receive training in dealing with epilepsy.	Two or three carers' files of carers linked to clients with special needs
	Carers given training about clients' individual special needs (eg sign language, special diet) as required.	Consumer telephone survey
	75%+ of client families report that they are satisfied that their carer is sufficiently well trained.	Survey

Managing good practice 12

The aim of this section is to give an overview of some of the thorny issues that managers and scheme coordinators have to address. These include:

- budgets;
- payments;
- complaints;
- equipment;
- legal liability;
- tax/social security;
- managing waiting lists;
- workloads.

Introduction

Within any scheme there will be a number of areas which loosely constitute 'management'. The responsibility for these will vary depending on the nature and location of the scheme, but it would be good practice for the scheme coordinator to know what areas are covered and where responsibilities lie.

This section is designed to highlight some key issues and to look at minimum responsibilities. It is only an introduction and will be developed over time.

Budgets

It is the responsibility of any service to draw up a budget adequate to its needs. This also serves to demonstrate actual costs to interested parties. Within family-based schemes the largest costs will be staffing and payment to carers. Staffing levels will be decided by local indicators (see workload section, page 147) and carers' payments should be set within nationally recognised bands. The last national survey of family-based short-term care services in the UK (Prewett, 1999) highlighted wide variations in payments to carers.

Setting a budget

The following may need to be considered:

- **Medical fees:** check financial arrangements with panel medical advisor.
- **Payments for carers:** which may increase in line with inflation.
- **Recruitment of staff:** this will need to be written into any contract in the case of voluntary organisations.
- **Staff salaries:** with 'on costs' to cover National Insurance.
- **Staff subsistence/mileage etc:** to cover expenses.
- **Public transport:** cab service or an allowance for transport costs.
- **Carers' training:** to cover all costs from training materials to attending the Shared Care Network conference.
- **Staff training:** though some may be free locally.

- **Recruitment of carers:** including leaflet/ newspaper advertising etc.
- **Insurance:** to include building and contents as well as cover for carers.
- **Cleaning:** for office cleaning and maintenance.
- **Rent**.
- **Council tax/water bills**.
- **Electricity/gas/telephone** (or a proportion in shared accommodation).
- **Office equipment/stationery:** to cover not just basic stationery but computer maintenance and so on.
- **Photocopying/postage**.
- **Carers' equipment:** health and safety equipment and domestic equipment.
- **Translation costs:** to cover all translating and interpreting costs.

For voluntary agencies which need to budget for all costs there will be numerous other headings, including Heating and Telephones, through to Equipment and Insurance.

Good practice is not about defining set budgets but for each scheme to be sure its budgeting fully reflects the costs of schemes. As value for money indicators enter all services, there needs to be clarity when setting budgets as to who is provided for, at what cost, with what results. The unit-costing of services has already arrived and services need to be sure they can meet 1989 Children Act regulations within a reasonable cost band. Budgets need to take account of the extra administrative and social work costs associated with implementing the 1989 Children Act regulations.

Complaints

The management of complaints procedures is an integral part of good practice. Complaints procedures need to be open, available and easily accessible to all members of the community (see the end of Section 9 on **Reviewing the approval of carers**). However, a telephone survey of carers carried out by Shared Care Network in 1997 found that only 43% of carers knew about a complaints procedure (Newitt et al, 1997).

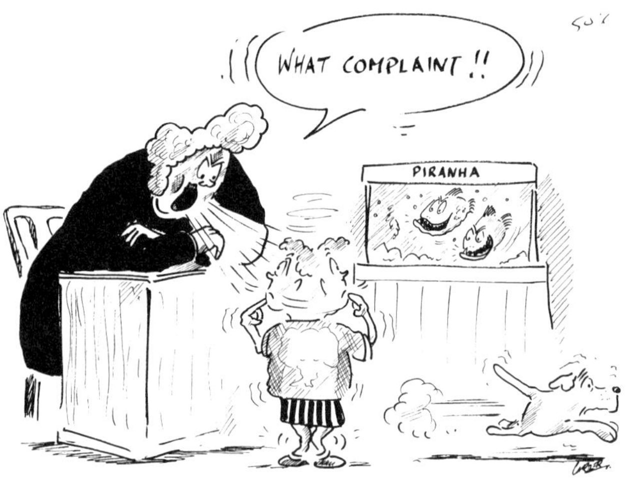

All complaints, both informal and formal, should be monitored at management level with care being taken to note any emerging trends. In services which deliver practical support to families, complaints tend to be lower than in other services because families fear they will jeopardise their entitlement to the service if they do complain. This should not lead to complacency. We should instead encourage carers and families to speak up, if they have any reservations about what is on offer from the agency. While complaints may be difficult to deal with at the time, they almost always lead to an improvement in practice standards.

Health and Safety

Since the first edition of *Stronger links*, issues around health and safety for both carers and children have become increasingly important. Booklets in the *'In safe keeping'* series, to be published in 2000 by Shared Care Network, address the areas of health and safety for carers, safe care and moving and handling. Below are a few specific issues you will need to consider.

Equipment

Schemes have a responsibility to ensure the health and safety of children placed with carers. As a minimum, this should mean a health and safety checklist during the carers' assessment, prior to approval, and the supply of basic equipment once the child is placed. The most common of these items include stairgates, socket covers, cooker guards, fire guards and so on. All equipment should carry current British Standards markers. Where more specialist equipment is required, for example, bathing aids, these should be discussed with a physiotherapist/ occupational therapist known to the child before any equipment is provided. If specialist equipment is needed it may be worth checking if there is a local joint equipment store where items may be loaned (health or social service physiotherapists will know of this).

Some schemes now make the installation of particular health and safety equipment a requirement. The most common of these relate to fire safety. Services need to be clear about their position on smoke alarms/fire blankets and be consistent about the application of any requirements that exist.

Legal liability

The world of legal insurance remains complex. However, the basics for schemes remain that short-term carers are clearly foster carers under the 1989 Children Act. They are performing a task delegated to them by the council, and therefore should be insured while carrying out that task.

Insurance covers a number of areas in relation to damage caused by children placed. Legal liability, however, relates to the cover for carers should they need recourse to law, for example, if they are prosecuted for negligence, or involved in child protection procedures. Schemes do not need to delve into the world of legal liability but should be clear what cover carers have under the scheme's insurance policy and should issue accurate advice accordingly. So:

- check with the local fostering service and ensure short-term carers have the same cover as foster carers;
- be clear what the council limitations are;
- if you are concerned, ring specialist agencies like National Foster Care Association and seek further advice.

Carers should receive all insurance information in writing and in a way which makes it accessible and straightforward.

There are specific legal issues which apply to children with complex healthcare needs. These have been fully covered in *Towards a healthy future* (Servian et al, 1998).

Tax

Income tax procedures vary across the country as local Inland Revenue offices reach local agreements. Again, good practice may be about negotiating with the Inland Revenue, but may equally be about being clear about what your local arrangement is. In some parts of the country there is a nil tax payment for short-term carers, whereas, in others, up to 33% of payments are deemed as taxable.

It is important, particularly for carers who work, that schemes are clear about their local tax agreement. This needs to be issued to carers in writing as part of a carers' pack.

If you don't know what your local tax agreement is:

- check with the fostering department;
- check with the local Inland Revenue office;
- ring Taxaid (see **Useful organisations** at the end of this guide).

Social security

Many of the short-term carers recruited by schemes may be on Income Support or other state benefits. The rules on tax and insurance also apply to them.

!

Be clear about your position

Put it in writing

Currently, social security is covered by Income Support (General) Regulations, Schedule 9, para 26. This states that families who take on the care of a child who is not a member of their family, but lives with them temporarily, and who are paid by recognised agencies, will not lose any of their benefit. However, the introduction of the Jobseekers' Allowance has made this position less clear. It is suggested that you seek local advice.

Managing waiting lists

Nearly 90% of schemes surveyed in 1999 have a waiting list. The average number waiting was 27 children. Nearly half the children awaiting a link were waiting nine months or more (Prewett, 1999).

One of the biggest challenges confronting schemes is children who wait. In managing a waiting list (as opposed to just having a waiting list) practitioners need to ask themselves key questions:

- Are there any children who will never be placed?
- Are there some children who could be placed with a targeted recruitment campaign?
- Are there some children who would benefit from more flexible arrangements, for example, Saturday day care or in-home care, and can it be provided?
- Are there some children referred even though in the assessment family-based short-term care is not in their interest?

Good practice is not about providing all things to all people. It's about being clear about your skills, abilities and limitations.

Once the questions about children on waiting lists are addressed, it may be the case that some are turned down for the service. This may be harsh, but to leave children waiting forever is less desirable.

All children on waiting lists should be monitored and reviewed internally every six months. The purpose of monitoring is to be clear why children wait, what reasons stop them being linked and to look at emerging trends. Family-based short-term care schemes within any locality act as key information collectors and providers for children with disabilities. Any information about trends on waiting lists may provide an essential input into the development of other services. Some children may wait simply because there is a four- or six-month wait for an assessment. Good practice will not solve a shortage of resources but it will at least identify and clarify why children wait and help provide a case for improving service delivery.

A recent ombudsman's ruling in 1998 concerning Surrey County Council and a child who had been assessed as eligible for a service which he/she did not receive, has implications for the management of individual care for children for whom a full assessment has been conducted. This reinforces the need to be honest with families at the outset about the constraints under which your scheme operates and the likelihood of appropriate matching. All information passed to families should also be communicated to the agency professionals and reiterated at the six month review.

Workloads

The issue of what constitutes a 'full caseload' for family-based short-term care scheme workers is a long-standing one.

Much of the debate centres on the issue of work with children and families. At one extreme, workers may be involved exclusively with recruiting and supporting carers with no direct work with the families and children. At the other extreme, scheme staff may be expected to take on the full statutory responsibilities for children. Neither of these options is ideal and there clearly needs to be a balance.

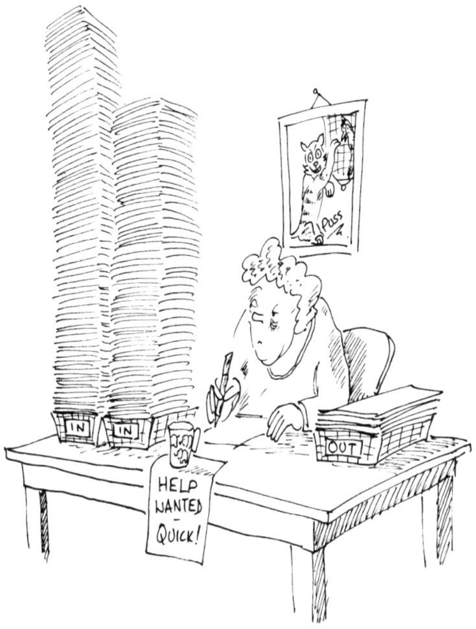

It is important in any scheme that workload arrangements are discussed and that the responsibility for children is clarified. It is a myth to believe that all children with disabilities will have an allocated worker (and they may not need one) but major change in the lives of children or their families is unlikely to be best served within the confines of short-term care. This is particularly important for voluntary agencies because they need to be clear which delegated responsibilities they are carrying out and where their input in children's lives begins and ends.

In terms of numbers and workloads the nearest estimate we have comes from the Audit Commission report, *Seen but not heard* (1994), which recommends, for short-term fostering, a limit of 20 carers per worker. This does not include a large element of children's work and, on this basis, short-term care scheme workloads should not be significantly greater than this.

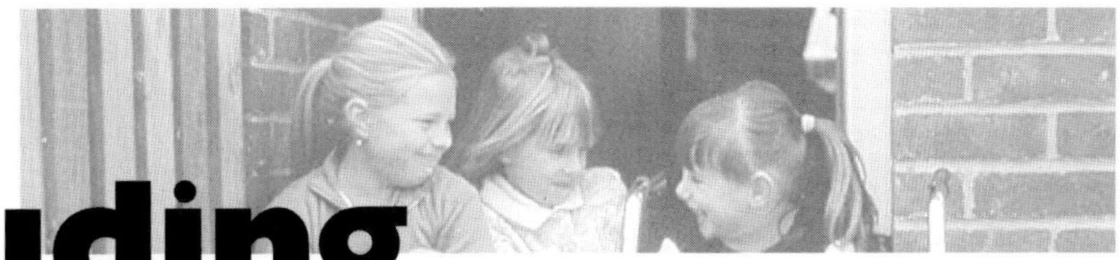

Concluding comments

The guidelines offered in this book are intended as suggestions for good practice and not prescriptive statements. Not all aspects of running a family-based short-term care service will have been covered and there may be questions which remain unresolved.

The guidelines should be of use not only to workers setting up new schemes but also to workers on established schemes who can measure their own practice against the good practice offered.

It is acknowledged that practice changes, and *Stronger links* is intended to be a living document which will be adapted and updated regularly. If there is any aspect of practice that you feel needs to be addressed and is not included in this guide, let us know – contact Shared Care Network in Bristol and the national coordinator will bring it to the attention of the national committee.

This is the first amended version of *Stronger links*, which is the first national good practice guide to be produced for family-based short-term care schemes. By coordinating and improving standards, family link schemes can begin to assert the important position they occupy in the whole range of provision that supports families.

Policy statements

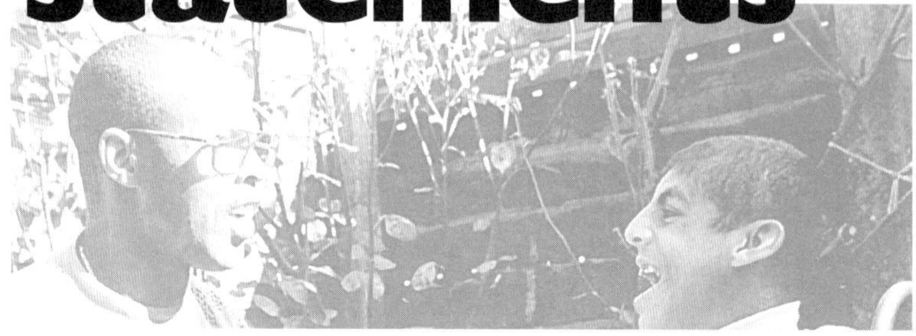

The aim of this section is to tackle some of the difficult issues which services find themselves facing. These issues have been brought to the attention of the Shared Care Network Policy Advisory Group who have put together the following statements. The policies are produced as a result of consultation with the Shared Care Network membership via the national newsletter.

The areas which the group have focused on so far which are included in this second edition are:

- moving and handling;
- equal opportunities – carers, children and families;
- same-race placements.

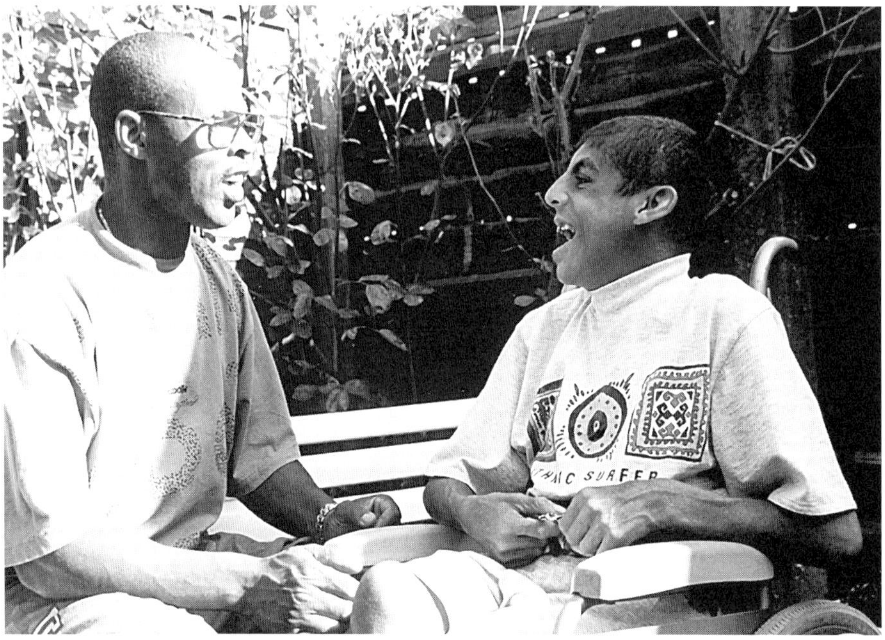

The EC directives on moving and handling: Background information and guidelines for implementation

Moving and handling – why is this important?

The Department of Social Security estimates that 81 million days of incapacity were lost due to back pain in 1992, with the highest incidence among the 16-44 age group. Anyone offering care to someone who needs to be lifted or turned regularly will be especially vulnerable. Clearly, many family-based short-term carers are at risk of back pain and the EC directives on moving and handling have raised some important questions for carers. The regulations also state that employing authorities must have a moving and handling policy in place.

Legislation and guidance

The legislation the EC looked at included:

- *1974 Health and Safety at Work Act;*
- *1992 Manual Handling Operations Regulations;*
- *1992 Management of Health and Safety.*

There are differing interpretations of the legislation. If your local authority classes carers as employees then Section A applies.

If your authority does not regard carers as employees then the legislation does not apply, but the guidance in Section B is suggested as good practice.

Section A – where employing authorities consider carers to be employees

What the regulations mean for users and their families, carers, professionals and employing authorities.

Service users

Users require a comprehensive risk assessment carried out by an appropriately qualified professional.

Support carers

- **Assessment of carer's environment:** the carer's environment has to be inspected in order to check its suitability for the individual. This should be carried out by an appropriately qualified professional.
- **Training:** carers must receive training in moving and handling from an appropriately qualified professional. This training should enable them to perform all the tasks required and would involve a step-by-step breakdown of all handling activities involving the individual in their care. These instructions should be documented as part of the placement agreement (contract) and agreed.
- **Insurance:** should cover any eventuality that may occur while the individual is with the carer and their family.

Scheme organisers

Scheme organisers should be responsible for:

- ensuring that a risk assessment of the individual and carer's environment has been carried out by someone who is suitably qualified;
- ensuring that initial and specific training for carers has been arranged and carried out by the appropriate professionals;
- ensuring that this is documented as part of foster care agreements and agreed by the carer and agency;
- ensuring that specific instructions/standards are maintained via regular updating and review;
- facilitating adequate insurance cover for the carer, individual and themselves.

Employing authorities

The legislation requires employing authorities to provide assessments of the host carer's environment and the needs of each user. Authorities are also required to provide training in moving and handling for carers. The employing authority is responsible for ensuring that all safety checks and assessment procedures have been carried out. It is recommended that local authorities employ suitably qualified professionals, for example, occupational therapists, to assess the environment and the needs of the service user.

General issues to be considered

- Scheme organisers need to be alert to the feelings and needs of the user's family.
- The legislation requires an 'inspection' of people's homes and they may be required to make changes to their homes and/or have equipment installed. Scheme organisers should aim to minimise the intrusion to the support carers and their families. A checklist should be drawn up by an expert to prepare carers for likely changes.

These issues should be raised, discussed and agreed and subsequently included in any moving and handling policy.

Section B – where employing authorities do not consider carers to be employees

Where link families are providing short-term care on behalf of the local authority but are not employees the Manual handling Operations Regulations (1992) do not apply. However, the local authority retains duties under Section 3 of the Health and Safety at Work Act (1974) to ensure, so far as reasonably practicable, the health and safety of non-employees who may be affected by the department's undertaking. The following is suggested good practice.

Service users

As part of a child assessment it is important to look at their moving and handling needs. These needs should be identified and recorded.

Support carers

During assessments carers should:

- be encouraged to think about what sort of children they could offer care to, taking into account manual handling issues and the physical environment in which care would be offered;
- be offered training in manual handling techniques – as a minimum this could be a basic group training run by an appropriately qualified professional;
- have insurance cover for any eventuality that may occur while the individual is with the carer and their family.

Scheme organisers

The person making the arrangements for the placement should ensure that the child is safe. Scheme organisers should therefore take responsibility for ensuring the following:

- that the child's needs are considered and that they are matched with an appropriate family and environment including possible problem areas relating to access, for example, differing internal levels and structures should be noted and included in the social worker's assessment;
- that training for carers has been made available;
- that this is documented as part of foster care agreements and agreed;
- that the child's moving needs have not changed, via regular updating and review;
- that adequate insurance cover for the carer, individual and themselves has been arranged.

Employing authorities

Employing authorities have duties under the Health and Safety at Work Act (1974) to carers (see page 154). The following is suggested as good practice in order to enable this:

- that employing authorities make available resources to scheme coordinators in order for them to arrange appropriate training;
- that employing authorities provide adequate insurance cover for the carers, users and workers;
- it would be good practice for schemes to have an allocation in their budget for equipment – health authorities and social services may also wish to pool resources and negotiate access to an equipment store.

If you are unsure about your authority's position regarding the status of carers, it is recommended that you write to both your authority and local health and safety officer. When ascertaining their position, it is suggested you make clear that if you do not receive a reply you will assume that carers are classed as employees, and that you will, as far as possible take the appropriate steps.

Shared Care equal opportunities – carers, children and families

Equal opportunities practices for recruitment, staff development and so on have already been established. Shared Care Network would want to ensure that the principle of equal opportunities is extended to the children, families and carers with whom it works.

Legislation and guidance

The principles of the 1989 Children Act are central to the work we undertake. There are certain relevant points regarding equal opportunities:

- *the child's welfare is paramount;*
- *we must work in partnership with families, carers and children;*
- *consideration should be given to the child's religious, racial, cultural and linguistic needs;*
- *carers should reflect the community we serve.*

Likewise, the 1990 NHS and Community Care Act highlights features which should shape the way our services are delivered, including:

- *individual assessments and plans;*
- *services adapted to meet individual needs;*
- *greater choice and flexibility;*
- *packages of care.*

Principles relating to equal opportunities

Principles are commonly held beliefs about the kind of society we wish to see and how people would be treated in it. Shared Care Network is committed to the principle of equal opportunities. We acknowledge that some groups in society face discrimination and are disadvantaged on the grounds of gender, race, disability, religion, age and sexuality. Shared Care Network is working to counter such discrimination in all its activities.

Our statement of belief

Shared Care Network values the contribution of all members and sections of society and would seek to promote and encourage their participation in the development of services.

Shared Care Network will challenge attitudes and practices which directly contravene the beliefs of an individual or which constitutes any behaviour that is racist and/or discriminatory.

Putting principles into practice

Service provision should reflect relevant legislation and good practice. In order to ensure that we work in partnership with children, adults, their families, current and prospective carers, consideration should be given to the following:

- Schemes should ensure that their premises and carers' homes are accessible to people with a disability: they should alert their local authority/ organisation where there are issues of access, for example, offices, community resources, which would impede a person's ability to take part in any proceedings relating to them.

- Service users and their families should be actively encouraged to participate in shaping the way their services are organised by, for example, making good reciprocal links with organisations within the community.
- Information should be provided which is communicated in a way that is easily understood and accessible.
- Services should be designed which offer individual choice and options and are able to respond to requests for help. Applicants should be given a clear expectation of services and the available resources. Carers should be representative of the multi-racial, multi-cultural society in which we live.

It should be acknowledged that every person with a disability has a right to an advocate and schemes should be actively encouraging this by:

- raising users' awareness of this service;
- encouraging carers where appropriate to become advocates;
- use of professional/voluntary advocacy services;
- recruitment, training and assessment of carers should reflect this equal opportunities statement by ensuring that the approval/reapproval panels are adequately trained and made up of a cross-section of the community;
- schemes should ensure that parents, users and carers are aware that they have the right to complain; if a complaint procedure is available a copy should be given to all appropriate persons.

Shared Care same-race placements

Legislation and guidance

The 1989 Children Act Guidance and Regulations suggest that:

A child's ethnic origin, cultural background and religion are important factors for consideration. It may be taken as a guiding principle of good practice that, other things being equal and in the great majority of cases, placement with a family of similar ethnic origin and religion is most likely to meet a child's needs as fully as possible and to safeguard his or her welfare most effectively. (1989 Children Act Guidance and Regulations, Vol 3, Section 2.40)

Introduction

Shared Care Network is highlighting the needs of black and minority ethnic individuals by promoting short-term placements which reflect their cultural, racial and religious identity. This principle applies in the same way to white individuals for short-term placements.

During the 1960s and 1970s the prevailing attitude was that colour was unimportant and that placement of black children with white families was the way to achieve an integrated society. Although well meaning, this attitude was, on the whole, unhelpful, because it implied that cultural and racial differences were superficial and that provision did not need to be varied for different ethnic communities. During the 1980s people began to recognise the individual needs of children from black and minority ethnic groups.

Black and minority ethnic groups are severely under-represented as short-term carers and users. In their 1993 study, Beckford and Robinson found that of the 8,000 short-term carers (children's schemes) then in the UK, only 6% were from black and minority ethnic groups and only 8% of the estimated 16,000 users were from these groups.

Why same-race placements?

There are many reasons why a same-race placement is important. Black children and their families are subject to not only overt racism but also to the subtle negative images of black people that society continues to generate. Children easily internalise these negative stereotypical images and it is therefore important to counteract them by providing positive black role models.

Race is at the core of an individual's identity and its importance cannot be overestimated. The cultural needs of children and adults with disabilities have traditionally been seen as coming second or not at all. Culture is, however, at least as important for people with the most severe disabilities as it is for people with no disabilities.

People with severe disabilities communicate their needs to the world through their senses, hearing, sight, touch, taste, smell, and these images are often culturally related. The following example illustrates this point.

Amir is a Bangladeshi Muslim child of 12 who has profound cerebral palsy and is blind. He is most responsive to his own cultural triggers, the feel of a sari, the sound of his own language, the smell of his own home and the taste of familiar food. Imagine the confusion caused to this child if placed in an environment where these cues were not available to him.

Good quality short-term care is about ensuring continuity for a child between his or her own home and placement: familiarity is comforting to most people. Where a child has limited communication it is essential. One cannot measure the confusion caused to a child when this is not possible.

These issues should apply to all services whether they have one black user or many black users.

Putting principles into practice

The role of the link social worker/scheme coordinator

In order to offer the best service to children and adults we must recognise and respect their cultural and religious needs. When matching children and families, the child's culture, race, language and religion should be considered. Good planning is essential to meet the needs of children and this includes training. Workers should explore not only formal sources of training, but also use the strengths of the particular communities to help them understand their culture. By building relationships with local communities and gaining trust, workers are also more likely to encourage the recruitment of new carers within these groups.

Schemes need to ensure that they have carers who represent fully their local communities. The recruitment of black carers is discussed in Section 1, **Publicity and recruitment**, page 15.

Black children need the survival skills to develop a positive racial identity. Shared Care Network believes that the best way of doing this is to match children of particular creeds and cultures with families who share the same beliefs, and this should always be the primary aim.

Partnership with parents

Partnership with parents is one of the key principles of the 1989 Children Act and should be a significant factor in planning a placement for a child. Where a family cannot be found which exactly meets the child's cultural and religious background, the parents should be consulted to find out which aspects of the child's culture they consider to be most significant in creating a match.

Of equal importance are the wishes of the child. The child's views should be sought regarding their placement and if the child has difficulty communicating the needs, innovative methods should be employed to enable them to have a voice (see Section 6 on **Consulting children, parents and carers**).

What about parents who say they don't want a same-race placement?

The first thing you need to ascertain is why the parents feel that they do not want a same-race placement. Is it for any of the following reasons?

- They see white carers as superior due to internalisation of the attitudes towards black people caused by racism?
- They have previously had a poor experience of a same-race placement?

- They feel that placement with a family from their own ethnic group may affect their standing in their community?

It is important that these reasons are explored and that parents are offered a positive experience of care within their own cultural group.

Parents should be encouraged to meet a carer from their own ethnic group to discuss their anxieties before they make a final decision.

What about children of mixed parentage?

Children who have one white parent and one black will usually be regarded by society as black. They, too, therefore, need a positive black role model and should be placed in a family where there is at least one black adult.

What if a same-race placement isn't possible?

It is recognised that this may not always be possible. It is important to assess whether a more immediate placement with a family which does not entirely meet the child's cultural needs is preferable to a long wait for a very well matched family. In short-term family-based care the placements are planned and not usually made in an emergency, therefore it should be possible to find carers with the same or similar cultural background to their own.

Where placement with a family from the same cultural group is not possible it would be preferable to place the child with another black community rather than a white family. Although the support family may differ culturally they will have had similar experiences of belonging to a minority ethnic group in this country and they will almost certainly have experienced racism.

However, the issues around continuity of care remain. Where children and short-term carers do not share the same cultural and religious beliefs, carers should be fully prepared for the placement by:

- race awareness training – this should be a minimum requirement if a transracial match is planned;
- the support family must be able to accept the child as a black child in a positive way and not dismiss the child's colour or culture as insignificant;
- the family must be prepared to foster an awareness of the child's religious background;
- the family must be able to demonstrate their willingness and ability to differentiate between different life-styles, race and colour, without inferring the superiority or inferiority of one or the other;
- the child or children of the support family must be enabled to accept and relate meaningfully to the black child.

Throughout the preparation course and assessment, support families should be clear that once they accept a child and their family they are expected to respect that family's beliefs.

Support for short-term carers in transracial placements

Where a child has been matched to a support family from a different cultural group, the carers should be given full information about the particular child's religion and beliefs.

There are a number of resources to facilitate this in a clear and straightforward way. The Franklin Watts' *My belief* books look at belief through the eyes of a young child. The series includes:

I am a Jew

I am a Sikh

I am a Muslim

I am a Hindu

I am a Greek Orthodox

I am a Roman Catholic

I am a Buddhist

I am a Rastafarian

It should be made clear to short-term carers that if they have any difficulties in providing care that mirrors the child's cultural background that workers would be there to provide support and further information.

Summary

Shared Care Network actively promotes same-race placements which provide continuity between the child's own home and the short-term placement. This must always be our primary aim.

Where this is not possible, the child should be placed with another black community rather than a white family. Carers should be given race awareness training and full information on the child with whom they are matched including information on their beliefs. They should also receive full back-up and support. Carers should respect the child's cultural and religious needs and offer care that reflects this.

Services should be continually encouraging the wider recruitment of carers from minority ethnic groups. Only by ensuring that there is a sufficient pool of carers from these groups can services work towards same-race placements for the majority of children and adults.

References

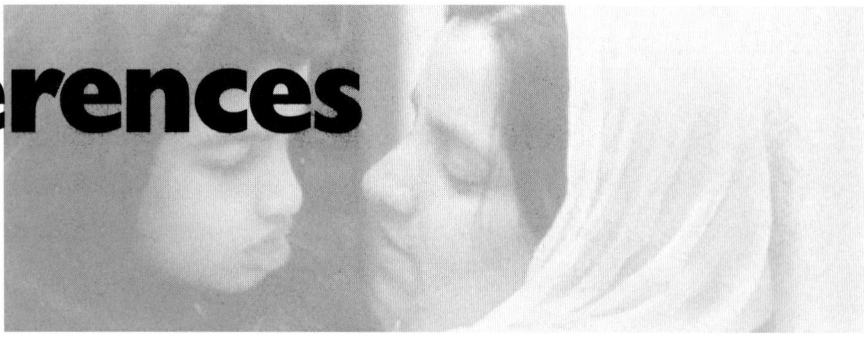

Aggarwal, M. (1984) *I am a Hindu. Gaytri devi goswami*, London: Franklin Watts.

Aggarwal, M. (1984) *I am a Muslim. Abu bakar nazir*, London: Franklin Watts.

Alderson, P. (1995) *Lisenting to children: Children, ethics and social research*, Basingstoke: Barnardo's.

Audit Commission (1994) *Seen but not heard*, London: HMSO.

BAAF (British Agencies for Adoption and Fostering) (1997) *Assessment Form F*, London: BAAF.

Beckford, V. and Robinson, C. (1993) *Consolidation or change? A second survey of family based respite care services in the UK*, Bristol: Shared Care UK, Norah Fry Research Centre, University of Bristol.

Burgner, T. (1998) *The Independent Longcare Enquiry*, Buckinghamshire County Council.

Cooper, C. (1985) 'Good enough, borderline and bad enough parenting', in M. Adcock and R. White (eds) *Good enough parenting*, London: BAAF.

Council for Disabled Children (1995) *Help starts here: A guide for parents of children with special needs*, London: National Children's Bureau.

De'Ath, E. (1982) *Establishing a true partnership between parents and professionals*, Parenting Paper No 6, London: National Children's Bureau.

DETR (Department of the Environment, Transport and the Regions) (1998) *Modern local government: In touch with the people*, White Paper M4014, London: The Stationery Office.

DFE (Department for Education) (1994) *Code of practice on the identification and assessment of educational needs*, London: HMSO.

DoH (Department of Health) (1998) *Modernising social services: Providing independence, improving protection, raising standards*, A White Paper, London: The Stationery Office.

DoH (1999) *Modernising health and social services: National priorities guidance 1999/00 – 2001/02*, London: DH Distribution.

Donnelly, H. and Horrex, W. (1995) *Respite care for children with autism: A survey of parents and a report of services available*, NE Essex Shared Care Scheme.

Griffith, A. (1993) *'When am I coming to stay?': A training pack for family link services for children with disabilities*, Cambridge: National Extension College/Shared Care[UK].

Health and Safety Executive (1974) *Health and Safety at Work Act*, London: HMSO.

Health and Safety Executive (1992) *Management of Health and Safety Regulations*, London: HMSO.

Health and Safety Executive (1992) *Manual Handling Regulations*, London: HMSO.

Kirkbride, L. (1999) *I'll go first*, London: The Children's Society.

Jones, V. (1989) *Quality indicators in family based respite care*, Unpublished.

Jones, V., Murphy, N. and Aspinall, V. (1997) *New horizons: Family based short breaks for people with autism*, Bristol: Shared Care Network.

Minkes, J., Robinson, C. and Weston, C. (1994) 'Consulting the children: interviews with children using residential respite care services', *Disability & Society*, vol 9, no 1, pp 47-57.

Morris, J. (1998) *Don't leave us out*, York: Joseph Rowntree Foundation.

Newitt, B. (1997) *A question of quality – Questionnaires and guidelines for telephone surveys of parents and link carers views in family based short term care services for children*, Bristol: Shared Care Network.

Newitt, B., Jones, V. and Robinson, C. (1997) *Quality counts – A review of quality assurance in family based short term care*, Bristol: Shared Care Network.

Preston, L. and Russell, P. (1997) *Positive partnerships in developing registers of children with disabilities*, Interim Report, London: National Council for Disabled Children.

Prewett, B. (1999) *Short-term break. Long-term benefit. Family-based short-term care for disabled children and adults*, Sheffield: Joint Unit for Social Services Research, Community Care.

Pugh, G. et al (1987) *Partnership in action: Working with parents in pre-school centres, Vol 1 and 2*, London: National Children's Bureau.

Robinson, C. and Stalker, K. (1992) *Why are we waiting? Reducing waiting lists: Practical guidance for developing short-term breaks*, London: HMSO.

Robinson, C., Weston, C. and Minkes, J. (1996) *Quality in residential short-term care services*, London: The Stationery Office.

Servian, R., Jones, V., Lenehan, C. and Spires, S. for Shared Care Network (1998) *Towards a healthy future: Multiagency working in the management of invasive and life-saving procedures for children in family-based services*, Bristol: The Policy Press.

Shared Care Network (1997) *After careful consideration .... An information booklet for panels assessing foster carers intending to provide short breaks for disabled children*, Bristol: Shared Care Network.

Shared Care Network (1998) *Policy group recommendations on the use of 'Looked after children' forms for children with disabilities*, Bristol: Shared Care Network.

Simons, K. (1993) *Citizen advocacy: The inside view*, Bristol: Norah Fry Research Centre, University of Bristol.

SSI (Social Services Inspectorate) (1994) *Services to disabled children and their families: Report of the national inspection of services to disabled children and their families*, London: SSI.

SSI (1998a) *Removing barriers for disabled children: Inspection of services to disabled children and their families*, London: DoH.

SSI (1998b) *Disabled children: Directions for their future care*, London: DoH.

Sturmey, P. (1993) 'The readability and human interest of information leaflets from major British charities: an unintelligible boring replication?', *Mental Handicap Research*, vol 6, no 2, pp 174-83.

UK Joint Working Party on Foster Care (1999a) *UK National Standards for Foster Care*, London: NFCA.

UK Joint Working Party on Foster Care (1999b) *Code of practice on the recruitment, assessment, approval, training, management and support of foster carers*, London: NFCA.

Utting, Sir William (1997) *People like us – The review of safeguards for children living away from home*, London: The Stationery Office.

Ward, L. (1997) *Seen and heard: Involving disabled children and young people in research and development projects*, York: Joseph Rowntree Foundation.

Acts

Department of Health (1986) *Disabled Persons (Services, Consultation and Representation) Act*, London: HMSO.

Department of Health (1989) *Children Act*, London: HMSO.

Department of Health (1990) *National Health Service and Community Care Act*, London: HMSO.

Department of Health (1991) *The Children Act (1989), Guidance and Regulations, Vol 6, Children with Disabilities*, London: HMSO

Department of Health (1991) *The Children Act (1989), Guidance and Regulations, Vol 3, Family Placements*, London: HMSO.

Department of Health (1994) *1991 Registered Homes (Amendment) Act*, London: HMSO.

Department of Health, Looking after Children Project (1995) *Good parenting, good outcomes*, London: HMSO.

Department of Trade and Industry (1984) *Data Protection Act*, London: HMSO.

Useful organisations

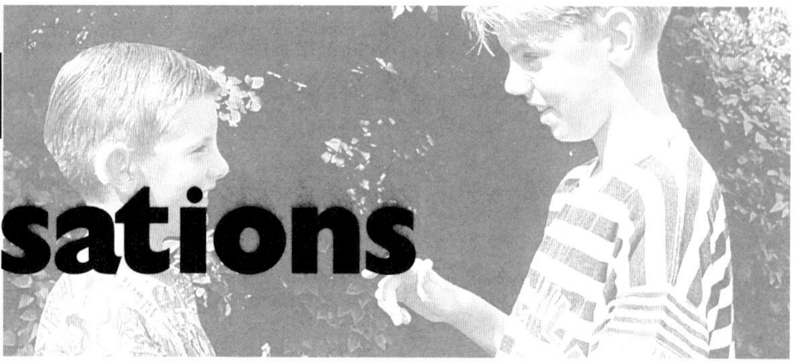

BAAF (British Agency for Adoption and Fostering)
Skyline House, 200 Union Street, London SE1 0LX;
Tel (0171) 593 2000; Fax (0171) 593 2001

Barnardo's
Tanners Lane, Barkingside, Ilford, Essex IG6 1QG;
Tel (0181) 550 8822; Fax (0181) 551 6870

BCODP (British Council of Disabled People)
Litchurch Plaza, Litchurch Lane, Derby DE24 8AA;
Tel (0133) 229 5551; Fax (01332) 295 580

Carers National Association
20-25 Glasshouse Yard, London EC1A 4JT;
Tel (0171) 490 8818; Fax (0171) 490 8824

Children's Legal Centre
University of Essex, Wivenhoe Park, Colchester, Essex
CO4 3SQ; Tel (01206) 873820; Fax (01206) 874 026

Citizen Advocacy Information & Training
162 Lee Valley, Technopark, Ashley Road, London
N17 9LN; Tel (020) 88804545; Fax (020) 8880 4113;
www.leevalley.co.uk/cait/

Contact a Family

170 Tottenham Court Road, London W1P 0HA; Tel (0171) 383 3555; Fax (0171) 383 0259; www.cafamily.org.uk

Cruse (Bereavement Care)

Cruse House, 126 Sheen Road, Richmond, Surrey TW9 1UR; Helpline (0181) 332 7227 (9.30am-5.00pm, Monday-Friday)

Disability Alliance ERA

1st Floor East, Universal House, 88-94 Wentworth Street, London E1 7SA; Benefits Advice Line (0171) 247 8763 (2.00pm-4.00pm, Monday-Wednesday)

Disabled Living Foundation

380-384 Harrow Road, London W9 2HU; Tel (0171) 289 6111; Fax (0171) 266 2922

Holiday Care Service (the UK's central resource on information about holidays for disabled and older people, one-parent families and those on low income)

2nd Floor, Imperial Buildings, Victoria Road, Horley, Surrey RH6 7PZ; Tel (01293) 774 535; Fax (01293) 784 647

Mencap Early Years Project

Mencap London Division, 115 Golden Lane, London EC1Y 0TJ; Tel (0171) 696 6918; Advice line (0171) 696 5581; Fax (0171) 696 5598

National Association of Adult Placement Services (NAAPS)
51A Rodney Street, Liverpool L1 9ER;
Tel/Fax (0151) 709 1200

National Autistic Society
393 City Road, London EC1V 1NG; Tel (0171) 833 2299;
Fax (0171) 833 9666

National Children's Bureau
8 Wakley Street, London EC1V 7QE; Tel (0171) 843
6000; Fax (0171) 278 9512

National Foster Care Association
87 Blackfriars Road, London SE1 8HA; Tel (0171) 620
6400; Fax (0171) 620 6401

NCH Action for Children
85 Highbury Park, London N5 1UD; Tel (0171) 226 2033;
Fax (0171) 226 2537

People First (promotes self-advocacy for people with learning difficulties)
Instrument House, 207-215 King's Cross Road, London
WC1X 9DB; Tel (0171) 713 6400; Fax (0171) 833 1880

PLA (Pre-school Learning Alliance)
69 King's Cross Road, London WC1X 9LL,
Tel (0171) 833 0991; Fax (0171) 837 4942

RADAR (Royal Association for Disability and Rehabilitation)
Unit 12, City Forum, 250 City Road, London EC1V 8AS;
Tel (0171) 250 3222; Fax (0171) 250 0212

Sense (the National Deafblind and Rubella Association)
11-13 Clifton Terrace, Finsbury Park, London N4 3SR;
Tel (0171) 272 7774; Text (0171) 272 9648; Fax (0171)
272 6012

Shared Care Scotland

109/111 Duncan Crescent, Dunfermline KY11 4DA; Tel (01383) 622 462; Fax (01383) 622 813

Shared Care Wales

Nuala Rawlins, 3-5 Bush Street, Pembroke Dock SA72 6X13

Social Policy Research Unit

University of York, Heslington, York YO10 5DD; Tel (01904) 433 608; Fax (01904) 433 618

Taxaid

(a charitable trust which provides free tax advice and assistance to persons in need and promotes public education in tax matters)
Linburn House, 342 Kilburn High Road, London NW6 2QJ; Tel (0171) 624 5216 (General Enquiries); Fax (0171) 624 5248

The Association of Crossroads Care Attendants Schemes Ltd

10 Regent Place, Rugby, Warwickshire CV21 2PN; Tel (01788) 573 653; Fax (01788) 565498

The Children's Society

Edward Rudolf House, 69-85 Margery Street, London WC1Z 0JL; Tel (0171) 841 4400; Fax (0171) 8414500

Values into Action

Oxford House, Derbyshire Street, London E2 6HG; Tel (0171) 729 5436; Fax (0171) 729 7797